"I feel like our souls wrote this book together, as I am so aligned with its message. I am privileged and honored to endorse it. It is a breathtakingly original mix of humor, radical wisdom, and new culture spirituality. Superbly written, easy to read, great stories, shatters the illusions that cause 'self abandonment,' and unwraps dynamics of freedom and security, the mystery of love relationships."

— Stan Dale, Founder of the Human Awareness Institute (HAI)

"No one can fully love until they are fully real. *Don't Be Nice, Be Real* takes important steps toward teaching us how to be real, and therefore how to love."

— Warren Farrell, Ph.D., Author of *The Myth of Male Power*

"This book is a must-read if you want to move beyond diagnostic categories, and toward the intimacy that comes from genuinely sharing your reality. Kelly Bryson speaks with authority about how to shift from angry defensiveness and control to relationships based on compassionate authenticity."

— Brad Blanton, Ph.D., Author of the Radical Honesty series

"*Don't Be Nice, Be Real* is probably one of the most authentic books about compassion and relationships I've ever read. For the first time ever, there is a book that stands apart from its competitors with its unique philosophy about compassionate selfishness. It may sound like an oxymoron, but believe me, it's not."

— Jennie S. Bev, Managing Editor of BookReviewClub.com

"Learning to speak my heart fully without blame or shame, and learning to reach into the experience of another through empathy — these have been two great gifts of Nonviolent Communication."

— Vicki Robin, Co-author of *Your Money or Your Life*

"In living the principles taught in this simple yet profound book, my life has dramatically improved. I now experience more harmony, more hugging, more laughter, and much more love! Kelly's style is hilarious and holy — and will convince readers of all ages of the spiritual practicality of putting oneself first."

— Diana Loomans, Author of *Full Esteem Ahead*

D0034416

"I found your examples and stories very helpful—they were specific enough that the abstract concept became a real experience. I enjoyed your word play (Cling-On, the Blame that Binds, Non-Rushin' Orthodox) and your humanness. You showed the readers you're just like us; we can relate to an author who hurts, says things he may regret, and dares to speak up to meet his needs. It is a book I'll recommend along with Rosenberg's when I am teaching and sharing Nonviolent Communication. When I'm in my accommodating mode, I feel the courage to speak up for my needs because you've showed me often in the book how it has worked."

—Moreah Vestan, Author of *Pleasures and Ponderings*

"Kelly Bryson wrote this book from the experience of a student and a teacher. His personal testimony shows how he walked for miles in 'nice' shoes, fell down emotionally, but picked himself up—eventually to help others. There are plenty of sample dialogs to train the reader for verbally expressing the way they feel, without fear of retribution. I recommend this book for all nice people who fear the word, 'No.'"

—Judine Slaughter, Editor, Express Yourself Books

"Just the title motivated me to order it, but when I went onto your website and read excerpts I was just blown away."

—Brother Dale Phillip, Self Realization Fellowship, Encinitas, California

"Thanks for taking Morrie's inspiration to heart."

—Mitch Albom, Author of *The Five People You Meet in Heaven*

"If you are tired of being one of the 'nice dead people' in the world, buy this terrific book."

—Lawrence Carter Sr., Ph.D.
Founder, Gandhi Institute for Reconciliation

"I really loved your book. I like the way it expressed the Passion side of NVC just as Marshall emphasizes the Compassion side. I love the way it focuses on the importance of being true to oneself first and then we can have compassion for others."

—Wes Taylor, Nonviolent Communication Trainer, Flagstaff, Arizona

"The book inspired me immensely. It's dense with nuggets of different subtleties of the dance of human hearts."

—Stuart Watson, MPA, Coordinator
Oregon State Network for Compassionate Communication

"You are truly a master in your ability to teach empowering communication in any situation. Your workshop opened the door to authentic communication within our department. We now have much more understanding of what is working and what is not working with the communication between team members. You are awesome!"
— Ken D. Foster, Manager Tony Robbins Research International, Inc.

"Thank you for writing your book! I was very touched by your sense of humor, vulnerability and your incredible stories — they definitely sparked some personal healing insights for me. I have been recommending the book to lots to friends, colleagues and coaching clients as one of the best personal growth books I have read in a long time."
— Jacqueline Peters
Coaching and Facilitating for Insights that Lead to Results

"I am excited by all the ways you are spreading Nonviolent Communication. I have begun reading your book and have recommened it to many others."
— Sylvia Haskvitz, Nonviolent Communication Trainer, Tucson, Arizona

"I am enjoying reading your book. I am recommending it to my friends. The more books like this that are available, the easier my work as a trainer becomes."
— Mel Sears, Nonviolent Communication Trainer, Seattle, Washington

"I found Chapter 15, 'Beware Of Nice Therapists' inspiring. It is helping my friend Mary write her dissertation on mental health at the community level and Nonviolent Communication."
— Dunia, Nonviolent Communication Trainer, Africa

"Thank you for the joy of reading *Don't Be Nice, Be Real.* I enjoy the tone — your recommendations of things to do to spoil a relationship I find hilarious — and the personal experiences you share. It meets my need for companionship and fun, and helps me to identify feelings that I drowned in an upbringing based on fear, guilt and shame."
— Inge Brink, Nonviolent Communication Trainer, Denmark

"This book is so full of clarity and fun. It reaffirms all I have been learning and teaching in Nonviolent Communication, with new insights galore! Thank you heaps!"
— Martine Algier
Nonviolent Communication Trainer, San Francisco, California

"I enjoyed reading your book and found it valuable in enhancing my consciousness of Nonviolent Communication. Your examples, perspective and presentation offered many fresh insights that deepened my understanding."

—Gregg Kendrick
Nonviolent Communication Coordinator, Charlottesville, Virginia

"Thank you for writing this powerful book. I stayed up most of the night reading it (laughing and crying out loud several times) because I want to read it at least twice before I meet with a particular client in about a week. I plan to buy as many books as I can and sell or gift them to my clients. I rarely have ever been so hungry for information—especially in the way that you share."

—Surrena Lovell-Hampton, Therapist

"I thank you for taking the time to write *Don't Be Nice, Be Real*. While reading this book, I connected with myself, my needs, and that part of me that is 'nice' and not 'real.' Your book gave me a deeper understanding of honoring my own self and needs first, which then allows me to give freely to others. A great deal of the anxiety I have suffered over the past five years is gone, and I feel liberated. Thank you for your love and generosity in helping others live their authentic lives."

—Mary Morgan
Nonviolent Communication Trainer, Orange County, California

"Just telling people the title stimulates a whole conversation in that it approaches Nonviolent Communication with backbone (I know I have one somewhere). With your help I'm able to relax and focus on needs and enjoy what life has in store. This is my way of living dangerously (on my way to greater honesty). Your personal experiences and breakthroughs followed by pointing out the principles involved helps me learn by example. It's like reading adventure stories."

—Tim Dolan, Nonviolent Communication Trainer, Montana Region

"I enjoy again and again how you bring so many of these modern 'disorders' in personal and social life to the 'simple' point of empathic communication, enlightening more and more not-so-well-known corners of myself. I sincerely hope your book will get widely distributed here in Germany and above all put into practice."

—Wilken Agster, Nonviolent Communication Practitioner, Germany

"I have been feeling scared, frustrated and hopeless, and reading your book is bringing me comfort and hope. Through your honesty I am supported in being more in my honesty. Through reading your experiences and insights, I am able to connect with my kindness for myself. I am beginning to validate my needs so I can be responsible for getting them met, and I then find it easier to feel compassion for my husband. I am grateful to have you and your book for support. I am starting to get what a huge difference this work is going to make in my ability to experience joy and love, and freedom from hurtful, painful behavior. The options that will become available to me are exciting."
— Rielle Pelletier, Therapist, Orange County, California

"So far I have bought three copies of your book. Although I try not to buy into Nonviolent Communication as a religion, I do use your book as part of my daily meditation. I want to invite my wonderful community of friends to experience an alternative method of communicating. Your book's title challenges the wimpy impression folks may have of compassionate communication. The step by step metamorphosis of your peace journey moved me to tears. It helps me see how to dance between real-life dialogue and under-the-hat work."
— Jeanne Smith, Teacher, Orange County, California

"Only when we understand how to be compassionate with ourselves can we offer compassion to others. In *Don't Be Nice, Be Real*, Kelly Bryson analyzes the obstacles that prevent this balance in our everyday lives."
— Gehlek Rimpoche, Author of *Good Life, Good Death*
Incarnate Lama of largest Tibetan monastery (Drepung Monastery)

"The values inherent in loving community are beautifully set forth in *Don't Be Nice, Be Real*. I bought several copies. My wife and I both think it is fantastic!"
— Matthew Bullock, Octogenarian Reader, Santa Barbara, California

"This book feels very authentic and close to life. It starts with examples of how to communicate nonviolently in our society, and moves toward a philosophy of utopia at the end. A German friend was very moved by reading just the first chapter. He could absorb no more, recognizing how he became 'nice' when staying at the home of his parents, who are dreadfully nice."
— Annette Deyhle, Ph.D., Scripps Institution of Oceanography

"Thanks for your great book and inspiration. What you have shared with me has been very, very important in working with my psyche. Everyone needs a copy of your book. I keep promoting it in my classes and online. One step at a time for humankind."

—Gururattan Kaur Khalsa, Ph.D.
Author of *The Destiny of Women Is the Destiny of the World*

"A moving and inspiring book. I love your personal sharings—it makes the content more real, and models showing one's vulnerability. The narrative is more story and less dry, overly-organized textbook. The first ten chapters cover sixteen core ideas of Nonviolent Communication. Chapters twelve through fifteen are each a world of healing—loved them!"

—Joel Rosenfeld, Ph.D., Professor of Psychology, Golden West College

"I am enjoying your book *Don't Be Nice, Be Real* very much. It is filled with deep insights and unusual ways of expressing ideas that grabbed my attention and made them really sink in. I just finished reading Dr. Marshall Rosenberg's book *Nonviolent Communication*. It complements yours very well. Dr. Rosenberg's book is written more from the perspective of the perpetrator, whereas yours is written more from the victim perspective. Both I can very well identify with. Thank you!"

—Gisela Sommer, Nutritionist, Orange County, California

"Kelly Bryson's particular gift is showing people how to communicate with others with clarity and compassion. I appreciate his loving and light-filled approach. His personal commitment to compassion and interpersonal harmony is inspiring."

—Rev. Kathy Hearn, Past President United Clergy of Religious Science

"Kelly Bryson is a sincere, honest, open-minded, compassionate, and creative communicator, with a wily wit. I honor Kelly for the wealth of experience he has gathered in Nonviolent Communication, and the way he has put his lessons together in *Don't Be Nice, Be Real*. Practicing the techniques in this book can move you out of old patterns and bring greater authenticity and aliveness to your life and relationships."

—Alan Cohen, Author of *The Dragon Doesn't Live Here Anymore*

Don't Be Nice, Be Real

Balancing Passion for Self With Compassion for Others

by

KELLY BRYSON, MFT

www.languageofcompassion.com

Published by
Elite Books
Santa Rosa, CA 95404
www.EliteBooks.biz

Library of Congress Cataloging-in-Publication Data:

Bryson, Kelly.
    Don't be nice, be real : balancing passion for self with
    compassion for others / by Kelly Bryson. --2nd ed.
    p. cm.
    Includes bibliographical references.
    ISBN 0-9720028-5-5

    1. Assertiveness (Psychology). 2. Self-actualization (Psychology).
    I. Title.
    BF575.A85B79 2004
  158.2--dc22
                                2004013814
Copyright © 2004, Kelly Bryson

The song "Covert War" on p. 12 is copyright © 1991 David Wilcox and is used
by kind permission of Irving Music, Inc., and Midnight Ocean Bonfire Music.

The following songs are copyright © 2002 Ruth Bebermeyer and are used with
her kind permission: "When I Come Gently" "Given To" "Words Are
Windows" "I Don't Want To Do That To Me Again" "I Can't Be in Touch With
You".

Nonviolent Communication(sm) is a service mark for the Center of the Center for
Nonviolent Communication, which may be reached at www.cnvc.org.

All rights reserved. No part of this publication may be reproduced, stored in a
retrieval system, or transmitted in any form or by any means, electronic,
mechanical, photocopy, recording, or otherwise without prior written permis-
sion from Sparrowhawk Publications, with the exception of short excerpts used
with acknowledgement of publisher and author.
Cover by Victoria Valentine
Interior design by Authors Publishing Cooperative
Typeset in Skia and Book Antigua
Printed in USA
Second Edition

10 9 8 7 6 5 4 3 2 1

CONTENTS

Foreword 10

Acknowledgments 11

1. Don't Pay the Price of Being Nice 13

2. Perfecting Your Selfishness 37

3. Feeding Your Attention Hog 45

4. Filling the Hole in the Soul 55

5. The Duty Giver 59

6. Confessions of a Cling-on 67

7. Do You Want to Be Right or Have Meaningful Relationships? . . 77

8. Healing the Blame that Blinds 87

9. From Fighting Fair to Fun Fighting 97

10. The Ecstasy of Empathy 135

11. The Danger of Deserve 155

12. The Myth of Motivation 161

13. Compassion Under Fire — Hot Talk in Hot Spots 183

14. Becoming a Non-Rushin' Unorthodox 217

15. Beware Of Nice Therapists 231

16. Our Culture Doesn't Work Anymore 251

17. Creating the New Culture 295

The Author and His Work 329

Foreword

by Marshall R. Rosenberg, Ph.D.
Founder, Center for Nonviolent Communication

In one of my favorite plays, "A Thousand Clowns," the lead character Murray tells the social workers who have come to force his nephew to attend public school, "Before I give him over to you I want to make sure he won't learn how to become one of the nice dead people. I want to be sure he'll know when he's chickening out on himself." I believe "nice deadness" is the result of the education necessary to maintaining a Dominator economy and culture. Kelly Bryson's book gives practical tools for recognizing when we are "chickening out" on ourselves and for bringing ourselves back to life. In his humorous way, Kelly gives examples and techniques for applying Nonviolent Communication to connect compassionately with ourselves and others.

Kelly's book shows that as we affirm the beauty of our own needs we greatly increase our power to meet the needs of others with great joy. It also describes concrete, masterful ways to negotiate our needs with caring, compassion and consideration for others.

In the play, Murray goes on to tell the Powers that Be: "I want him to get to know exactly the special thing he is or else he won't notice it when it starts to go. I want him to know the subtle, sneaky, important reason he was born a human being and not a chair." None of us will know that special thing we are as long as we allow the fear of conflict to keep us hiding behind our "mask of nice." The principles and skills of Nonviolent Communication described in the book can help us overcome that fear and begin to experience that subtle, sneaky, important meaning of being authentically and divinely human. And as we embrace this authentic divinity more and more, we can contribute to creating a culture of compassion that can truly serve us all.

Acknowledgments

First and foremost I would like to acknowledge my spiritual partner Debbie. I appreciate her patience as I spent so many late night hours at the computer, her support in both hearing and reading my ideas ad nauseam, her consistent, complete, compassionate caring for our daughter Mataya, and her total caretaking of the household so I could write. I also appreciate her steady stream of warm affection, understanding, and courage in the crazy times.

I acknowledge my little Mataya, who some day will be able to read this, for all the loving, sparkling, refreshing energy her presence provided me in play breaks from my hours of writing.

I am forever grateful for tons and tons of inspiration, love, direction, understanding, wisdom, modeling, and attention from my precious teachers. I have special appreciations: Dr. Marshall Rosenberg for teaching me how to "perfect my selfullness" in a way that increases my contribution to others; the late Virginia Satir for seeing me as her "Wonderful One"; John Bradshaw for helping me heal from my childhood wounds; Stan Dale for helping me see the divine nature of my potency; Danaan Parry for inspiring my inner "Warrior of the Heart"; Robert Johnson for helping me "own my gold"; Param Hans for showing me the power of "satsong," Rollo May for inspiring my own "courage to create"; Dr. Deborah Taj Anapol for expanding my mind; and Riane Eisler for showing me the profound importance of restoring respect for the feminine.

I am grateful to all the people who have been in my trainings and sessions: you have been my life-blood. By allowing me to give to you, you helped me experience my purpose for being, an intoxicating energy of healing and wholeness, a renewal of spirit, and a crucible for my own growth.

Although I have tried to give credit to Marshall Rosenberg throughout the book where it was due, I am sure there are phrases, principles, concepts and maybe even stories that originated with Marshall for which he was not acknowledged. Because I have been studying with him for over 20 years, there is a bit of blur as to the origin of many ideas expressed in this book.

Marshall Rosenberg has shared his personal self with me, heart and soul, his genius and experience. He has touched me deeply and I have been transformed. How can I express my gratitude?

How does a flower thank the sun for the warmth and light that has opened it?

Chapter

DON'T PAY THE PRICE OF BEING NICE

You better not shout, you better not cry,
You better be nice, I'm telling you why...

Have you been a naughty or a nice boy or girl? You have been nice? Well, then you must be enjoying the rewards of being a good little boy or girl. These rewards often include depression, intermittent explosiveness, career confusion or job meaninglessness, ambiguous anxiety, low awareness of one's own needs, either flat or explosive relationships, resentment about being the victim of "mean people," subtle self-hate and assorted psychosomatic illnesses.

What a tragedy that our culture puts us in conflict with our human nature. It took me till the end of the school year in first grade before I could sit for the whole period with my hands folded, my feet together and my mouth shut. Then I was told "What a nice little boy you were today!" That is when I was seduced into the slavery of people pleasing. I prostituted my own essence and prevented my little boyness from expressing itself in order to get those few little drops of perverted praise.

The energy it took to control such a vital force took a noticeable toll on my physical body. One of my mentors, Virginia Satir, noticed it the first time she met me. She put her hand on my uptight shoulder and proclaimed to a large audience of people in La Jolla, California, "Now this man has paid a heavy price for being nice. In order to survive, he has learned to be a people pleaser, and now carries all this tension in his shoulders in order to control his spontaneous expression." This was powerful news coming from Satir, who is a mythic figure in the social science and mental health fields. She is called the Mother of Family Therapy and is credited with coining the term "people pleaser." John Bradshaw, best-selling author and creator of the popular Public Broadcasting Service series "Bradshaw on the Family," and other well known self-help authors, draw heavily on her work. And she was right. Not only had I paid a heavy price, but so had everyone around me.

So now I am trying to get the word out that being nice has its price. I've already told you some of the "rewards" the nice person receives. Here are just a few of the costs that the nice person's family, friends, and associates pay:

1.   Always being nice prevents people around the nice person from receiving feedback that would stimulate their growth. By "growth" I mean gaining knowledge about, and insight into, oneself and others.

2.   Nice people often react with pain if anyone around them expresses uncomfortable feelings. They get angry, thinking others should have to be nice too. Or they feel hurt and confused if someone does not appreciate their niceness. Others often sense this and avoid giving them feedback, thus not only effectively blocking the nice person's emotional growth, but preventing risks from being taken. You never know with a nice person if the relationship would survive a conflict or angry confrontation. This greatly limits the depths of intimacy. And would you really trust a nice person to back you up if confrontation were needed?

3. With nice people you never know where you really stand. The nice person allows others to accidentally oppress him. The nice person might be resenting you just for talking to him, because really he is needing to pee. But instead of saying so he stands there nodding and smiling, with legs tightly crossed, pretending to listen.

4. Often people in relationship with nice people turn their irritation toward themselves, because they are puzzled as to how they could be so upset with someone so nice. In intimate relationships this leads to guilt, self-hate and depression.

5. Nice people frequently keep all their anger inside until they find a safe place to dump it. This might be by screaming at a child, blowing up a federal building, or hitting a helpless, dependent mate. (Timothy McVeigh, executed for the Oklahoma City bombing, was described by acquaintances as a very, very nice guy, one who would give you the shirt off his back.) Success in keeping the anger in will often manifest as psychosomatic illnesses, including arthritis, ulcers, back problems, and heart disease.

Proper Peachy Parents

In my work as a psychotherapist, I have found that those who had peachy keen "Nice Parents" or proper "Rigidly Religious Parents" (as opposed to spiritual parents), are often the most stuck in chronic, low-grade depression. They have a difficult time accessing or expressing any negative feelings towards their parents. They sometimes say to me "After all my parents did for me, seldom saying a harsh word to me, I would feel terribly guilty complaining. Besides, it would break their hearts." Psychologist Rollo May suggested

-§-
Emotionally
starving children
are easier to
control; well fed
children don't
need to be.
-§-

that it is less crazy-making to a child to cope with overt withdrawal or harshness than to try to understand the facade of the always-nice parent. When everyone agrees that your parents are so nice and giving, and you still feel dissatisfied, then a child may conclude that there must be something wrong with his or her ability to receive love.

I remember a family of fundamentalists who came to my office to help little Matthew with his anger problem. The parents wanted me to teach little Matthew how to "express his anger nicely." Now if that is not a formula making someone crazy I do not know what would be. Another woman told me that after her stinking drunk husband tore the house up after a Christmas party, breaking most of the dishes in the kitchen, she meekly told him, "Dear, I think you need a breath mint." Many families I work with go through great anxiety around the holidays because they are going to be forced to be with each other and are scared of resuming their covert war. They are scared that they might not keep the nice garbage can lid on, and all the rotting resentments and hopeless hurts will be exposed. In the words to the following song, artist David Wilcox explains to his parents why he will not be coming home this Thanksgiving:

Covert War
by David Wilcox

Dear mom and dad here's why I can't come home.
I can talk with either one of you just fine, when it's either one alone.
But Thanksgiving table's goin' to be pulled out bigger.
If we talk at all, one of you will pull the trigger.

I used to run those battle lines try'n to smooth over what got said.
Try'n to get a medal, try'n to get some shrapnel in my head.
Thought it was my duty to plead and to implore,
But I caught too much crossfire in your covert war.

Television talk fills the air so you don't have to start.
You claim your territories in the rooms upstairs,
To keep yourselves apart.
Holy days they bring us all together,
After so much left unsaid.
You taught us well not to kick under the table.
Kick under your breath instead.

I love you and I'd never want to see you bleed
When comments cut like steel

> So to hold your fire I'd block the shot and
> Take the hit for you as if I could not feel.
> I thought they passed right through me
> And I had no scars to hide.
> Now I open up and try to love
> And find they're still inside.
>
> 'Cause I used to run those battle lines
> Trying to plead, to implore.
> Please won't you hold the cease-fire out a little longer
> 'Till the next uproar.
> I took it all in childhood
> But I can't take it no more.
> 'Cause I caught too much crossfire in your covert war.

There is a huge difference between someone who has true respect, honor, and empathy for the needs of others and someone who is "nice" because they were trained to honor the needs of others and not their own. For the most part, observing the behavior of both of these people one might come up with the same evaluation; that they are polite, cultured and have good manners.

But the intention, the feeling and the reasons behind these same behaviors are totally different. The "nice" person is operating from conventional morality, which is what child psychologists Kohlberg and Piaget call Stage Three of Moral Reasoning: "Good boy or nice girl orientation." This is where "right action" is behavior carried out to please or impress others. The genuinely empathic and considerate person operates from what Kohlberg and Piaget call Postconventional Morality. They tell us that this level is usually reached only after age twenty, and even then, by only a small portion of the adults in our culture. It is called "postconventional" because the moral principles that underlie the conventions of a society are actually understood.

How important is it to teach children to be considerate of others through their own understanding and from their own autonomous free wills? How important is it that children develop empathy and compassion—and not just learn to be good or nice? Alfie Kohn makes this dramatic point in his great book *Punished by Rewards:* "Autonomy is not simply one value among many that children should acquire, nor is it simply one technique for helping them grow into good people. In the final analysis, none of the virtues, including generosity and caring, can be successfully promoted in the absence of choice. A jarring reminder of that fact was provided by the following declaration made by a man whose name is (or should be) familiar to most of us: he recalled being taught that the highest duty was to help those in need, but he learned this in the context of the importance of "obeying promptly the wishes and commands of my parents, teachers, and priests, and indeed of all adults.... Whatever they said was always right."

The man who said this was Rudolf Hess, the infamous commandant of Auschwitz, the German death camp. Prosocial values are important, but if the environment in which they are taught emphasizes obedience (being nice because the teacher will punish you if you aren't and reward you if you are) rather than autonomy, all may be lost. Jean Piaget, the world's best-known expert on children's developmental stages, author of *The Moral Judgment of the Child,* put it simply: "Punishment...renders autonomy of conscience impossible."

Anyone want to help me start PAPA, Parents for Alternatives to Punishment Association? (There is already a group in England called 'EPPOCH' for end physical punishment of children.)

In Kohn's other great book *Beyond Discipline: From Compliance to Community,* he explains how all punishments, even the sneaky, repackaged, "nice" punishments called logical or natural consequences, destroy any respectful, loving relationship between adult and child and impede the process of ethical development. (Need I mention Enron, the Iraqi Abu Ghraib prisoner abuse scandal or certain car repairmen?) Any type of coercion, whether it is the seduction of rewards or the humiliation of punishment, creates a tear in the fabric of relational connection between adults and children. Then adults become simply dispensers of goodies and authoritarian dispensers of controlling punishments. The atmosphere of fear and scarcity grows as the sense of connectedness that fosters true and generous coopera- tion, giving from the heart, withers. Using punishments and rewards is like drinking salt water. It does create a short-term relief, but long- term it makes matters worse. This desert of emotional connectedness is fertile ground for acting-out to get attention. Punishment is a use of force, in the negative sense of that word, not an expression of true power or strength. David R. Hawkins, M.D., Ph.D. author of the book *Power v. Force* writes "force is the universal substitute for truth. The need to control others stems from lack of power, just as vanity stems from lack of self-esteem. Punishment is a form of violence, an ineffec- tive substitute for power.

Sadly though, parents are afraid not to hit and punish their chil- dren — for fear they will turn out to be bank robbers. But the truth may well be the opposite. Research shows that virtually all felony offend- ers were harshly punished as children. Besides children learn thru modeling. Punishment models the tactic of deliberately creating pain for another to get something you want to happen. Punishment does not teach children to care about how their actions might create pain for another; it teaches them it is ok to create pain for another if you have the power to get away with it. Basically might makes right. Punishment gets children to focus on themselves and what is happen- ing to them instead of developing empathy for how their behavior affects another.

Creating "Correct" Children In the Classroom

One of the most popular discipline programs in American schools is called Assertive Discipline. It teaches teachers to inflict the old "obey or suffer" method of control on students. Here you disguise the threat of punishment by calling it a choice the child is making. As in, "You have a choice, you can either finish your homework or miss the outing this weekend." Then when the child chooses to try to protect his dig- nity against this form of terrorism, by refusing to do his homework, you tell him he has *chosen* his logical, natural consequence of being excluded from the outing. Putting it this way helps the parent or teacher mitigate against the bad feelings and guilt that would otherwise arise to tell them they are operating outside the principles of compassionate relating. This insidious method is even worse than out-and-out punishing, where you can at least rebel against your punisher. The use of this mind game teaches the child the false, crazy-making belief that they wanted something bad or painful to happen to them. These programs also have the stated intention of getting the child to be angry with himself for making a poor choice. In this smoke and mirrors game, the children are "causing" everything to happen and the teachers are the puppets of the children's choices. The only ones who are not taking responsibility for their actions are the adults.

Another popular coercive strategy is to use "peer pressure" to create compliance. For instance, a teacher tells her class that if anyone misbehaves then they all won't get their pizza party. What a great way to turn children against each other.

All this is done to *help* (translation: compel) children to behave themselves. But of course they are not behaving themselves: they are being "behaved" by the adults. Well-meaning teachers and parents try to teach children to be motivated (translation: do boring or aversive stuff without questioning why), responsible (translation: thoughtless conformity to the house rules) people. When surveys are conducted in which fourth-graders are asked what being good means, over 90% answer "being quiet." And when teachers are asked what happens in a successful classroom, the answer is, "the teacher is able to keep the students *on task*" (translation: in line, doing what they are told). Consulting firms measuring teacher competence consider this a major criterion of teacher effectiveness.

In other words if the students are quietly doing what they were told, the teacher is evaluated as good. However my understanding of "real learning" with twenty to forty children is that it is quite naturally a bit noisy and messy. Otherwise children are just playing a nice game of school, based on indoctrination and little integrated retained education.

Both punishments and rewards foster a preoccupation with a narrow egocentric self-interest that undermines good values. All little Johnny is thinking about is, "How much will you give me if I do X? How can I avoid getting punished if I do Y? What do they want me to do and what happens to me if I don't do it?" Instead we could teach him to ask, "What kind of person do I want to be and what kind of community do I want to help make?" And Mom is thinking "You didn't do what I wanted, so now I'm going to make something unpleasant happen to you, for your own good to help you fit into our [dominance/submission based] society." This contributes to a culture of coercion and prevents a community of compassion. And, as we are learning on the global level with our war on terrorism, when you use your energy and resources to punish people, you run out of energy and resources to protect people. And even if children look well-behaved, they are not behaving themselves. They are being behaved by controlling parents and teachers.

My little three and a half year old came home from her private, insanely expensive, super spiritual progressive preschool with a very long face and no energy to play with me. I asked her what was going on. With her usual dramatic flare, swaying arms hanging down and a frown to the ground, said "They maked me do things." with a tone of lifelessness. I asked her what she meant and she explained that the teacher's helper had been grabbing her arms and pulling them to her sides explaining that "We keep our hands to ourselves in class." I went to the class to observe and sure enough, often when one of the children would touch another child the teacher's aid would gently pull their hands back explaining that we must keep our hands to ourselves. I am sure that it had never occurred to the aid that *she* was not practicing what she was preaching and was missing an important opportunity to have a respectful dialogue about how we want to treat each other.

Dr. Piaget confirmed that true moral development and self-responsibility can only occur where the child is surrounded with moral behavior and allowed to grow her own understanding of the ideals of integrity, interdependence and interconnectedness. He put it this way, "Moral autonomy appears when the mind regards as necessary an ideal that is independent of all external pressure."

But this moral autonomy is not supported in our topsy-turvy school and family systems, where respect for authority actually means fear of authority. Where there is fear there cannot be respect. Although a child may envy or fear the power a parent or teacher wields over them, their feelings do not include the sacred, essential quality of loving reverence that makes respect, respect. It is akin to the battered dependent wife saying she loves and respects her abuser, when her daily experience is fear. Jerry Jampolsky, author and founder of the Center for Attitudinal Healing, reminds us that it is fear, not hate, that is love's opposite.

If, however, a truly educational atmosphere is created based on respect for autonomy instead of intimidating indoctrination, children can then deeply understand that rules are needed to maintain the social order. They do not have to be obeyed out of a blind acquiescence to authority, but are followed on the bases of mutual agreement. At the same time, the needs of the individual are protected and respected.

Nice "Guise" and Gals

It is at this Stage Six—Universal Ethical Principle Orientation, of Piaget's that people make moral decisions based on self-chosen ethical principles that are applied in consistent ways. So although both may not cheat at cards, the "nice" guy does not cheat because he wants people to like him. The "real" guy does not cheat because he senses the interconnectedness of life and all beings, and wants to contribute to the harmony and well-being of all. He has consciously chosen to live by certain principles that selfishly keep him in harmony with himself, his community, nature and life. Living by these principles keeps him free from resentment. He is full of the self-worth that comes from receiving feedback that he is serving the life within himself, his community and nature.

This is not the case for "nice" guys. (And by "nice guys" I don't mean the *real* nice guys like the one just described, but someone motivated by an agenda, or fear. Someone for whom being nice is a put-on role, a "Nice Guise" if you will.) Nice guys and gals not only finish last, they do so with great resentment. They then turn this resentment inwards (because it would not be nice to express it) and become depressed.

I work with a lot of divorced, depressed, disillusioned women who tell me "It's not fair. I did everything right, touched all the bases and I have nothing to show for it. Now I don't even know who I am or what I want." This is because our culture did its job well with these women. Sadly, our culture is designed particularly to make women keenly aware of what others want, at the expense of an awareness of their own needs. In fact, submissiveness for women is romanticized and eroticized. Think of all those images little girls are exposed to so early on in their lives they have no way to defend themselves: images of Prince Charming sweeping her off her feet (removing her from her foundation — the Earth) and riding off with her to his castle; images of a husband carrying her over a threshold into their new, happy life; images of her father giving his daughter (like a piece of heirloom furniture) to the groom; to images of the caveman dragging his woman by the hair. (Off to the cave to have sex with her.)

In so many fairy tales, like Cinderella and Sleeping Beauty, the only thing the hero knows about the girl is that she is beautiful. He shows no interest in her intellect or personality — or even her sexuality. The man is either a ruler or has the magic power to awaken her, and all she can do is hope that her physical appearance fits the specifications better than the other girls. In the original Cinderella story, the stepsisters actually cut off parts of their feet to try to fit into the glass slipper. Maybe this marks the origins of the first cosmetic surgery.

Besides romanticizing Cinderella's misery, the story also gives the message that women's relationships with each other are full of bitter competition and animosity. The adult voice of womanly wisdom in the story, the stepmother, advises all her girls to frantically do whatever it takes to please the prince. This includes groveling, cutting off parts of themselves, and staying powerless.

I was heartsick to watch Disney's "The Little Mermaid" with my three-year-old daughter. The little mermaid agrees to give up her voice for a chance to go up on the "surface" and convince her noble-man to marry her. She is told by her local matron sea witch that she doesn't need a voice — she needs only to look cute and get him to kiss her. And in the story, it works.

These are the means to her one and only end: to buy a rich and respected guy. Women are taught to listen only to an outside patriar-chal authority. No wonder there is so much self-doubt and confusion when faced with the question, "What do *you* want out of your life?"

This question alone can be enough to trigger an episode of depres-sion. It often triggers a game of Ping-Pong in a woman's head. Her imagination throws up a possibility and then her pessimistic shotgun mind shoots it down. The dialog may look something like this: "Maybe I want to go back to school.... No, that would be selfish of me because the kids need me.... Maybe I'll start a business.... No I hate all that dog-eat-dog competition.... Maybe I'll look for a love relation-ship.... No, I am not sure I am healed yet...." and on it goes.

Nicenecks

A part of me is concerned about introducing yet another label into the culture, but sometimes the potential fun outweighs the danger of contributing to people's stuckness. So my new label (with apologies to comedian Jeff Foxworthy who warns us "you just might be a redneck if...") is "Niceneck." A "niceneck" is someone who is too nice for their own good. Or maybe I should invent a disease out of it like "nice-neckism." Or maybe ADDS (Assertiveness Deficit Disorder Syndrome) and open up treatment centers all over the country to help people recover from it. I could model them after all Codependency Treatment Centers. I will create a list of symptoms that everyone can relate to, like occasional restlessness with life, loneliness, and intermit-tent depression — and then suggest that I have the cure. Here is a checklist to help decide whether you are a "niceneck" and need to put yourself on the waiting list to check into one of my marvelous new ADDS treatment clinics (after they get built and if you have insurance.) You just might be a "niceneck" if:

1.   When someone bumps into you from behind with their grocery cart, you apologize.

2.   People have a tendency to grab you by the shoulders and shake you a lot.

3.   Some Babble-onian (that's someone who uses more words than you know how to enjoy hearing) has been talking to you forever on the phone but you are afraid to tell them you want to go to sleep. You are afraid of either hurting their feelings (which really means that you are afraid of feeling guilty) or being perceived as rude.

4.   You have trouble saying real "Yes's" and "No's" i.e. ones that you really mean.

5.   You are constantly thinking about how to say things without upsetting people.

6.   It takes you an hour to tell the telemarketer you have no interest in buying a cactus ranch in Yuma. (Do you realize that you are the cause of the starvation death of the telemarketer's children? Because he could have made some money by selling to someone who was actually going to buy.)

7.   Your roommate skips out on you without paying his rent. Instead of filing in small claims court you spend hours meditating on the question, "Why did I create this in my life?" Or you may call and thank him for helping you face the karma of your money issues. This I would call graduate level Niceness: Avoiding Assertiveness through Spiritual Self-Blame, or AASS for short.

Now how did we come to be such aasses? One answer is that we were sweetly seduced by our teachers, parents and society with conditional love, bribes and punishments. I like the fun way Alfie Kohn says it in his book *Punished by Rewards: The Trouble with Gold Stars, Incentive Plans, A's, Praise, and Other Bribes:* "When we call out a hearty

'Good girl' in response to a child's performance, the most appropriate reply would seem to be 'Woof!' With respect to the workplace or public policy we talk casually about the use of 'carrots and sticks,' and there is food for thought here, too. Before these words came to be used as generic representations of bribes and threats, what actually stood between the carrot and the stick was, of course, a jackass."

And I doubt that it exactly inspires a love of learning that often teachers use extra classwork or more reading as one of their 'sticks.'

So we have all these nice parents out there trying to "do the right thing" by punishing and rewarding their children into becoming one of the nice dead people who create no problems for the social structure. Well meaning nice parents believe that it is necessary for their child's survival to learn to jump through hoops to respond to the rewards society has to offer. They have no idea how it deteriorates internal motivation to get their children hooked on external rewards. They make no distinction between self-esteem and esteem from others. They see no difference between celebrating one's accomplishments and contributions and constantly seeking external approval. I recognize that some of you are only aspiring "Nicenecks" perhaps because you have not been through the western punishment/reward school system, nor had other religious education that challenges you to mold yourself through self-disgust. If you want to catch up with the rest of us "Nicenecks" I suggest practicing the following:

Seven Steps to Self-Sacrifice (Or How To Become a Niceneck)

1. Listen to other people longer than you want to. Examples: Listen to telephone solicitors, religious missionaries, multilevel marketing acquaintances, and all your whining friends, to their satisfaction.

2. Do everything you feel obligated to do. Examples: Write thank you letters to all the relatives and acquaintances you think you should after each holiday. Go to every meeting, political rally or religious service you think you should. Contribute to every charity, and volunteer for every organization, that asks you for help. If no one asks, motivate

yourself to initiate a call to them. Live by the saying of famous TV counselor (although she has no degree in psychology) Dr. Laura: "Do the right thing." (I have this motto emblazoned on my very own $1.99 coffee mug, which Dr. Laura gave me for appearing on her show. Dr. Laura would probably feel better if she knew how guilty I feel, making fun of her motto after receiving that fine parting gift. I am still seriously appreciative that the Dr. Laura show paid for a stretch limo that brought myself and a friend from San Diego to Hollywood at a cost of about six hundred dollars each way.)

3. Work for a living, instead of figuring out how to get paid to play.

4. Do anything to prevent other people from freaking out.

5. Chant the mantra, "No pain no gain."

6. Adopt the motto: "Me last."

7. Call my aunt and volunteer to be her friend. She is a Jehovah's Witness, Amway salesperson, and black belt Babbleonian (meaning she can speak on the inhale as well as the exhale).

Look again at number three above, and consider the possibility of getting paid to play once you quit nicely conforming to the belief that "one must work for a living." I can tell you from my own real life that one does not have to do something unfun in order to survive financially. Sure, there are many sweat shop owners and proud McDonald franchise owners, who need nice dead people to fill their "McJobs". (Yes, mcjobs is now a word in the dictionary!) But the rest of us have become conscious of things we really enjoy doing and then figured out ways to get paid to do them. I love Marsha Sinetar's book *To Build the Life You Want, Create the Work You Love*. She tells the story of a woman who had fun receiving rapt attention from little children when she would read them a story. She developed a business called Traveling Storyteller. She dresses up in a white evening gown and sparkling tiara to tell stories to crowds of enraptured children near her home in New York.

How To Cure a Niceneck Through Nonviolent Communication

If none of the above steps to self-sacrifice appeal to you and you are tired of trying to get better at walking on eggshells, then I suggest walking in rhythm to the beat of your own soul and learning how to actually enjoy people freaking out about it. How? I teach Nonviolent Communication, a method of communication I learned from Marshall Rosenberg, its creator, to help myself with this.

When tempted to be nice and give up my needs I like to say, "I'm_____" followed by the emotional truth. For example, "I'm worried about staying on the phone with you because I want to get this article written before the deadline." Passion is the larger part of com*passion*. So I like to first have passionate self-compassion, fierce self-love, and then I can have compassion and empathy when others freak out. Then if my friend on the telephone line says, "Well fine, see if I ever call you again!" I can answer, "Are you hurt because you wanted to keep talking?" And if I can empathetically connect with her pain about wanting to continue connecting with me, I actually do enjoy the feeling of that connection. Also I can enjoy the sense of healing and relief it brings to that person to have her hurt truly heard.

Another way I enjoy people freaking out is when it gives me a chance to practice and celebrate my divine selfishness. For example, I once did an interview on a relatively big radio station that broadcast all over Los Angeles about using Nonviolent Communication in love relationships. I mistakenly gave out my home phone number during the show and consequently began receiving lots of calls at all hours of the day and night from lovesick men and women.

One morning at about 2 AM I received a call from what sounded like a crying teenager. I groggily answered with my usual self-programmed "Center for Compassion, Kelly Bryson speaking."

"My boyfriend won't answer my phone calls! What should I do?" said the tearful voice on the other end. I sleepily answered "You sound really hurt and upset."

"Yes I am! What should I do?" she sniffled.

"I'm sleepy right now, but if you wanted to call me back in the morning after 10 AM, I would be willing to talk with you."

"Never mind, I thought this was the Center for Compassion!" she said followed by the click of the line being disconnected. Her freak out gave me a chance to practice becoming inwardly conscious of my needs so that I can outwardly assert them when faced with a woman in pain (something I need practice in) and celebrating that I honor my self, my feelings and my needs. I went back to sleep with a warm guilt-less feeling of appreciation for myself.

Suppose your best friend asks you "Am I fat?" The nice friend would respond, "Oh, no! You're pleasingly plump."

The friend who is just learning tough love would say, "No, you are not fat. But your blood type is Ragu and you are outrageously obese, Mrs. Thunder Thighs, and I can no longer be involved in this friend-ship until you get into a treatment program."

The first response is likely to support your friend in rationalizing away a desire for a more healthy body. The second response would likely trigger a shame attack, necessitating a trip through the emergency room entrance to Baskin and Robbins (Basking in self pity and Robbin' themselves of health) for some Rocky Road Resuscitation. The nice friend's response is trying to meet the need for compassion and gentleness at the expense of honesty and trusting the other's strength. The tough love friend's response is a type of honesty, but at the expense of the gentle compassion needed to establish connection, which allows for lasting influence. This brutal honesty does sometimes influence the other to change out of shame, fear, hurt or guilt, but because it is coming from the outside and is pain-motivated, the change will likely be temporary. For change to be lasting, it needs to come from an inner willingness and be focused toward some pleasur-able goal like feeling alive and healthy. Pain is a good short-term moti-vator, but self-love or pleasurable satisfaction is necessary for sustained motivation.

If I want to be a lasting positive influence on my friend I need to come from gentle strength myself. In response to my friend's question "Am I fat?" I would give a Nonviolent Communication response: "Are you worried about your health or your attractiveness?" And then I would wait to give my friend space and time within which to be heard, to explore and unwrap what the issue is all about for her.

After she had received the empathy she needed I might then ask "Would you like to hear how I feel about your weight?" Again I would pause here to be sure she really was consenting and not just capitulating. (With certain friends, I have them sign a legal document in blood, stating that they truly do want my honesty, and that if my honesty messes up their lives, they will not complain to me about it.) It might sound like this: "I am very scared about your health because I want you for a friend for as long as I can have you. I am very sad that you haven't had a date in such a long time. I want you to be happy and have love in your life. How do you feel about what I am saying?"

In this world we are constantly faced with dealing with people who are consciously or unconsciously behaving in ways that can oppress us on some level. Many of our teachers taught us not to "talk back." We had to be quiet when our needs were not being met. We learned to deal with our pain by stuffing it, or taking it out on weaker beings. We learned creative ways to try to take care of our needs, like dissociating from them or using passive-aggressive tactics. By passive-aggressive, I mean what I taught myself to do in order not to risk getting punished for asserting my needs: I learned to pout. My internal dialog went, "I am hoping my pouting will make you so miserable that eventually you will come to me, guess what I need, and give it to me—without me having to go through the humiliation of asking for what I want."

To counteract these self destructive habits of either shutting down or acting out aggressively, I am teaching myself some new behaviors when someone else's behavior is not meeting my needs. Once I was in a workshop with Dr. Marshall Rosenberg, the founder of the international Center for Nonviolent Communication. I had just completed a huge piece of emotional work around issues related to my father. I had been crying in release — great belly sobs of grief — and I was now starting to catch my breath, as the focus of the group went on to the next person's issue. I unconsciously began to rock and make a little whimpering, squeaky sound on my breath's exhale. I was sitting right beside Dr. Rosenberg when he leaned over and whispered in my ear, so as not to embarrass me in front of the group, "That little sound you are making, is that soothing to you?"

I was startled from my self-involved state. "Ahh. yes," I replied.

"You know, Kelly, I'm really feeling irritated and frustrated right now," he said, "because I want to both comfort you, and be focused on this next person's issue. Could you find another way to soothe yourself?" I was a little embarrassed despite his consideration, but I was able to just open my throat a little more on the exhale and comfort myself through breathing and rocking. What Dr. Rosenberg demonstrated was three graceful steps to self-assertiveness:

1.   Demonstrating empathy for the feelings, needs and intentions behind the behavior. ("That little sound you are making, is that soothing to you?")

2.   Expressing our feelings and needs. ("You know, Kelly, I'm really feeling irritated and frustrated right now, because I want to both comfort you and be focused on this next person's issue.")

3.   Express a request for an action that demonstrates a willingness to get both people's needs met. ("Could you find another way to soothe yourself?")

Some Practice at Graceful Assertiveness

1.   Write down something someone did that was annoying to you, like they answered a cell phone call in a movie.

2.   Pretend you are speaking to this person and demonstrate non-judgmental understanding. Connect with that person by using the following form (you fill in the blanks): "Are you _____" (fill in a feeling like "worried") "because you_____." (Fill in a

want like, "because you want to make sure you don't miss an important call?")

3.   Pretend you then share your feeling, unmet wants, and your request: "I'm_____" (fill in a feeling like "worried") "because I_____" (fill in a want like "want to focus on the movie") "and would you be willing to_____?" (Fill in an action request like, "take the call outside?")

From Giving Up or Giving In to Giving To

The more I care about someone, the more painful it is to be "nice" to them or to allow them to accidentally oppress me. The other day my partner came bouncing into my room saying she was very hungry and asked if I wanted to go to breakfast. I really wanted to keep reading but I was too humble to admit that. I wish I had remembered what Golda Meir once said: "Quit being so humble; you're not that great." I chose instead to go to breakfast and subtly resent myself for giving up my need to read.

The tragic part of the story occurred a few days later when she once again asked me to go somewhere while I was reading. I felt the resentment rise up from my belly and a little voice saying, "I don't want to do that to me again." Then I felt the temptation to project the resentment, and blame her for asking. Finally I told her what was going on with me: I had given up my need for her sake the other morning. Immediately tears welled up in her eyes as she told me she never again wanted to be the stimulus for resentment or for me giving up my needs. Wow! I began to see, practically, how important it is not to be nice. When we sacrifice our needs for the other we can actually trigger pain for them. It is important to hang in there until we find win win solution. Whenever our niceness allows another to oppress us and prevent us from getting our needs met, we either resent ourselves, the other, or both. I would go so far as to call it a form of violence. It is the violence of self-abandonment, and whoever we allow to oppress us, we will subtly hate and withdraw from.

We are all taught that unselfish (translate "good"), flexible people know the value of compromise. Compromise, as I define it means, that we learn to share the resentment 50/50. Much compromise comes out of a scarcity consciousness that does not trust that we both could have all that we want. We fall back on compromise when we lack the energy and creativity to find the synergistic solutions that could get everyone's needs met fully. Compromise is a lack of trust in the compassionate generous nature of human beings that could lead to a shift that would allow for a true and natural "giving to" instead of a compromising resentful "giving in."

Unfortunately, our schools and families teach us to communicate in a way that makes compromise look like the best alternative. Unintentionally, our teachers and parents teach us to think and speak in terms of moralistic judgments, which highly increases the likelihood of conflict. And because these teachers and parents feel inadequate to negotiate potential conflict, they teach us the value of compromise. In cultures like ours, authority figures often think it is their job to teach us right from wrong, appropriate from inappropriate. Sadly, what we learn is to disassociate from our feelings and needs, and express ourselves in judgmental terms about what is wrong with other people. We learn to say things like, "It's not fair" instead of, "I'm hungry, would you share the donuts?" Or, "You're rude" instead of, "I'm feeling distracted, would you lower your voice so I can hear the movie?" Instead of gaining successful experiences of asserting our needs and getting what we want, we collect painful experiences. We ask for what we want in the only way we have been taught, through moralistic judgments of others, which gets perceived as an attack and provokes a counterattack. Then we not only don't get what we want, we end up feeling fear, shame and guilt. For example:

Jane: "You are afraid of intimacy and commitment" (a judgmental diagnosis instead of an expression of her own intimate feelings or requests).

John responds: "And you are needy and insecure. Get a life."

Or Little Jane: "You're mean. Why won't you let me play with you?"

Little John: "Because you are a little dweeb, that's why!"

No wonder we learn to stop expressing ourselves early on in life. We get so wounded by others' reactions to how we have learned to express our needs that we shut down. We learn: "If you are going to get along you have to go along."

This fear of not getting along with others is a primary driving force for the "Niceneck." This is because "Nicenecks" are terrified of being abandoned by others or being isolated from the group. This is partly why nice people deny that there is anything terrible going on, like in the Emperor's New Clothes story. To a niceneck it would be "rude" to tell a truth that might trigger discomfort for someone or to acknowledge that there is an elephant in the living room. (In my family there were herds of elephants being ridden by nude emperors parading through our living room.) You have heard the old saying "If you can't say something nice, better to say nothing at all." I have a new one "If you're going to say something nice better not to say anything at all."

From Sheeple to People

I suggest that the really catastrophic acts of violence in the world were passively condoned by the nice, educated, majority in the culture. In WW II, large numbers of people, particularly certain international religious leaders, knew what Hitler was up to and what was happening in the concentration camps but chose not to make waves. An elderly German statesman that I've studied with, Hans de Boor, told me that from his schoolroom they could smell the stench of burning flesh from the concentration camp extermination ovens outside their city. But the children told each other that this was just some new fertilizer plant. The Nazis were also trying to flee their inner demons and avoid the inner conflict created by German child-rearing practices. Manuals taught German parents to teach their children to "knock on the door to love through obedience to authority." This is why all they could do was be nice, go along, and never be naughty by saying "No!" to "Heil Hitler der Führer." It was out of this fear of coping with the inner conflict between their culture and their nature (inner child) that they supported their government in attacking what they were educated to believe was the "Evil Empire" out there. In this case it was the Jews.

Partly from my own experience in traditional schools, and partly from my reading of history, comes my distrust of traditional schools. Some say our public schools are doing what they were designed to do. Supposedly some factory owners got together in Lowell, Massachusetts, put some money together and asked their town council to create the first public schools in the USA, so they could get the docile, subservient workers they needed for their factories. I cannot help but wonder if early pharmaceutical companies also needed future Prozac users. Victor Frankel, MD, author of *Man's Search for Meaning* and originator of Logotherapy, shares my distrust as he makes even more troubling observations. He writes: "I am a survivor of a concentration camp. My eyes saw what no person should witness: gas chambers built by learned engineers, children poisoned by educated physicians, infants killed by trained nurses; women and babies shot by high school graduates. So I am suspicious of education! My request of teachers is: help your students to be Human. Your efforts must never produce learned monsters, skilled psychopaths or educated Eichmans. Reading, writing, spelling and arithmetic are only important if they serve to make students more Human."

In the foreword to this book, Marshall Rosenberg quotes Murray's words from the play by Herb Gardner *A Thousand Clowns*, about not wanting his nephew to become one of "the nice dead people" who don't know why they were "born a human being and not a chair."

I have been a good, nice useful chair for the society but it has cost me my creativity and my connection to my wild wonderchild. I'm relieved to report that this elan vital (vital life energy which cannot be created or destroyed) has not been murdered as I feared, but simply trapped in a tomb of fear, guilt and shame. As a recovering "Niceneck" I'm discovering and uncovering a long lost and precious friend of mine. Here is a poem I wrote to celebrate our reunion:

Homecoming
by Kelly Bryson

Heart broken by shattered childhood dreams.
Knowledge of Realms of Creativity lost,
I grieve the cost to my now lonely soul.
Panic is nearby, I want to fly, afraid to die.
But the Sirens of my Soul sweetly sing their song of loss,
And I want to hear, ignore the fear and allow my Self to
Come Home, come Home, ye who are weary come Home.
I relive the moment of our separation
and through this recreation
find my long lost soul again.
I start to feel my body soften,
resurrecting from its coffin
Of tension, armor and pain.
Oh great Joy, could it be, could it be?
That the soul I thought had been crucified,
Had just been lost, buried, and denied,
And is finally, finally reuniting with me.

Chapter

PERFECTING YOUR SELFISHNESS

I want to be very conscious of when it would be more gratifying to give to myself or to someone else. I cannot believe it, but just as I was writing the preceding sentence a dear friend came into my study and asked if I'd be willing to listen about some distress she was having. I am glad I was focused just on this line because I was able to tell her the truth, that it did not fit for me right now to give her my attention. I really wanted to continue giving to myself by writing this chapter. I was willing to allow her to suffer and trust that she could deal with her own pain. Because I said "No" to her, I won't be tempted to try to make her suffer later, when my anger about "giving in" resurfaces in the form of a punishing pout, sneaky sarcasm, or old fashioned blame and judgment.

I am confident that later I will really enjoy giving her my attention and she will sense that joy, which will help her trust that her need is really a gift to me. If I had given in, and given out of obligation or pity, she would sense and know it and possibly interpret herself as needy or burdensome to me. The octane of my attention will be much higher once I have taken care of my need to finish my thoughts. Then I can give to her in a way that she can trust she won't have to pay for later, and affirms that she is valued.

Here are three main blocks to asking for what you want:

1. Fear of hurting the other's feelings, i.e. fear of feeling guilty.

2. Not knowing you have permission to ask for what you want.

3. Fear of what you will tell yourself if they say "No."

Some people appear to be "super nice givers" but they are really focused on trying to buy love. They have very little connection with others, or true empathy for the needs of others. They are anxious to give so they can get feedback that they are liked. However, they are desperately focused on themselves and how to protect themselves from the inner voices that would say, "You're not nice enough. If you were, people would love you and you would feel okay about yourself." They are in a death raft in the middle of the ocean, drinking salt water, confused about why they still feel thirsty.

-§-
How can I show you that I value you without having to obey you?
-§-

Martyrdom is an ecologically bankrupt principle to apply in relationships. To the degree my partner Debbie sacrifices herself to try to care for our daughter, Mataya, she becomes emotionally, physically and spiritually depleted. From this depleted place she has less presence to give our daughter or anyone else. It never pays off to sacrifice, no matter how pure the intention to give seems to be. This is not the same as stretching to contribute to someone's well-being. But if what you are about to do is not solely and completely just for yourself, please don't do it.

Dr. Rosenberg was once watching his children blissfully feeding bread to some hungry ducks at the park. There was a profound quality of mutual giving between the children and the ducks. The children were grateful that the ducks were eating and the ducks seemed grateful to be fed. This quality of mutually selfish, yet satisfying, giving and receiving is what enriches relationships and people's lives. This quality keeps love growing and prevents the hardening of the heart's arteries known as resentment.

Dr. Rosenberg is fond of saying, "Please don't give me anything or do anything for me unless you can do so with the kind of joy a little child has when it feeds a hungry duck."

A short while ago my daughter Mataya fell asleep on my chest with her mouth nuzzled in my neck. Her sweet heaviness made it impossible for me to move. I thought about getting up to work, to do something useful that could help save the world. I told myself, "I should be writing my book, making progress, contributing." But her sweet heaviness kept inviting me into heavenly sleep with her. I reminded myself, "I am doing something, I am contributing. I am a fatherly futon for my child and that's what she needs right now. No, I can't fool myself. It's all for me. She's my little heroine and I am her addict. My mind is right, I should be doing something to save the world right now, but I am just not going to. I have no good excuse. I choose to abandon the world and indulge in the ecstasy of neck-nuzzling nectar."

And it may well be that holding my child and feeling that warmth and joy contributed more to the planet than making myself write my book from an attitude of obligation. Maybe it is what we are feeling that determines what consciousness and energy we are contributing to the planet. So maybe I did more to contribute to world peace by sunning myself on the beach with the sea lions, than I would have had I joined the very angry "peace marches" here in San Diego. (One of their slogans was "We're going to show San Diego what anger looks like!") I want to put my relationship with myself first, and getting stuff done second. Sure, I could make myself write a page, but then it's like cutting off the head of the goose that laid the golden egg. In other words, after I "make" myself do some writing, I might, out of resentment and protest make myself wait weeks before I am willing to write again. So I would like to place less importance on what I get done, and more importance on what energy I am coming from. If I get it done with fun, I won.

-§-
Greediness means that I quit denying myself the joy of high-octane giving.
-§-

If I "give in" to myself, I miss out on the opportunity to give *to* myself. I also give myself permission to "stay stuck" for as long as I want to. I reframe it as "sitting with my needs until I have more confidence that I am giving to myself" — not submitting to some part of myself. I want to give to both needs, just as a bird gives energy to both its wings in order to fly. Or as Plato says in *Phaedrus,* we have an earthly steed, representing practical bodily needs, and we have a heavenly steed, representing spiritual, emotional needs of the heart. The trick is to get them both pulling the chariot in the same direction, with our free will in charge.

Here are some mottoes to help you perfect your selfishness:

- Me, first and only, in every situation, at all times.
- Ask for 100% of what you want 100% of the time and be prepared to empathize with any response.
- Never listen to one more word than you want to hear from anyone.
- You never have to answer anyone's questions, because you are not on trial.
- Trust that all your needs are gifts to other people.
- Present your needs as if you were Santa Claus passing out gifts: "Ho, ho, ho you lucky dog, you get to give me a massage, if you'd like."
- Develop the willingness to *let* the people you love suffer (not to be confused with *making* them suffer).
- Never let anyone get his/her needs met at your expense. To do so is violence to both of you.
- Remember that when you are superficially nice, people do not respect you, they suspect you.
- Never do anything to prevent someone from freaking out (except babies under 15 months).
- Never give anyone the power to make you give in or rebel.

Adonis and the Hamburgers

Adonis, a fifteen-year-old "black male," leans over and whispers in my ear, "Kelly, there's only two hamburgers left and I want them both. What should I do?" My friend Adonis, plus ten other adolescent offenders, are having lunch at CATC, the Comprehensive Adolescent Treatment Center.

"Well Adonis," I say with caution, trying to stay a guide on the side, instead of a sage on the stage, "You know what I always tell you. Figure out what would be the most selfish thing you can do, and do that." Then, like the sun coming out from behind a dark cloud, a huge silly smile grows slowly across his face. He reaches down, grabs his fork, spears both of the remaining hamburgers, and plops them on his plate. He looks up toward me with the eyes of a returning hunter celebrating his kill. Then across the table comes a sour, matter-of-fact voice, "That's it, Adonis."

"What's it? What did I do?" says Adonis, moving quickly into his familiar defensive stance.

"That's it. You are not borrowing my skates tonight like you *thought* you were," says Jerry, Adonis's only semi-friend.

Adonis turns back toward me with genuine hurt and betrayal in his eyes. He says, "You set me up. I did what you said, acted selfish, and it didn't work."

"The problem," I replied, "is that you weren't selfish enough. You want the hamburgers and you want to borrow the skates tonight, right?"

"Right."

"So if you were thinking Big Selfish, your plan would have included the skates. I always try to get you to think like a Giraffe, looking at the Big Picture, from a very high perspective, right? So in order to keep being friends with Jerry and to still go for the hamburgers you might have asked, 'Does anybody else want another hamburger?'"

"I was too greedy," says Adonis as he returns the hamburgers to the serving plate.

"Expand your greediness to include taking care of your most precious resource, your good relations with other people."

Seeing the hamburgers returned to the status of community property, Jerry says, "That's okay, Adonis, I'm full, I didn't really want any more hamburgers anyway."

"Really!" says Adonis with childlike glee, "I can have both hamburgers? What about borrowing the skates?"

"Yeah, you can borrow the skates, just as long as you don't try to 'dis' [disrespect] me again," says the once again semi-friend.

"It works!" utters the amazed Adonis with exaggerated awe.

"Head"ing for Trouble

I have an acquaintance named Rex who occasionally becomes obsessed with hugging me. We were at a public workshop one day

-§-
Delaying
gratification
—Yuck!
-§-
Strategically
timing gratifi-
cation so as
to maximize
pleasure
—Yea!
-§-

when I heard him coughing and wheezing behind me. I moved to another seat. But that did not stop him. He began to pursue me, and did in fact finally corner me and hug me. I hugged him because I didn't want to trigger pain in him which he would then express in the community in the form of gossip. It was a mixture of my fear of creating enemies, being scapegoated, and financial fear. Instead of remembering to be selfish, I decided, "Okay, this situation calls for me to sacrifice my body and override my gut feeling to preserve the peace." I ended up with a horrible case of the flu.

As soon as I consider whether this situation might be one that calls for me to "go up to my head" to intellectualize with my brain instead of going with my gut reaction, to abandon my body, I've entered a realm of complexity and uncertainty. It's very similar to going to my head to think about a whether a situation calls for violence or not. If I'm not committed totally to looking for nonviolent solutions, no matter what, then the door of violence is always open to me. I'm always trying to decide if this person is a "good guy" and I should look for a nonviolent way of resolving the conflict, or a "bad guy" and it's okay to use violence.

If I think that it is *ever* okay to be violent with myself and abandon my body and my gut feelings for *any* reason, then I'm not committed to me. I can never really feel safe in the world if I can't trust that I'm totally committed to staying true to my guts.

I remember some of my first feelings of self-abandonment. It was when big people used to come up to me and rub my head and say things like, "He's so *cute!*" I hated it and yet for some reason I did little about it. Someone had taught me by age five that you must abandon your gut feelings when big people do things to you don't like. If I had listened to my body, I would have ducked or screamed, or pushed their hand away, or even said, "I don't like that." But I never did.

Until there is commitment to being true to one's body there is hesitancy and uncertainty. Until there's commitment, there is no tapping into the power and magic of providence. It can only come in to help when faith beyond reason is practiced. We have to step into the water before the seas part. I need to be willing to get into trouble if I am to avoid bigger trouble.

I had rather *you* be angry at me than *me* be angry with me. I'd rather get in trouble with you than with myself. If I stay true and connected with myself, then I have a chance to be present and work through whatever gets triggered in you. But if I abandon me, I can't deal with or be present to anything. Being nice depletes my energy, as I give it away to all the other nice, depressed, depleted people.

Just as feelings were once judged to be weakness, needs are often stigmatized as dependence, a lack of self-reliance, or an attempt at manipulation. The following chapters will show you how great an evolutionary — and revolutionary — step we take when we bring individual needs out of the shadows of shame and bring them into the divine light from which they came.

Chapter

FEEDING YOUR ATTENTION HOG

I was once at a New Age party and wanted to get the attention of some particularly lovely sari-wearing, belly-dancing women who were floating in and out of the various rooms. I had discovered that I could move past some of my fear and make a connection with people through singing. So I pulled out my guitar and started playing a song I had worked particularly hard to polish, Fleetwood Mac's "A Crystalline Knowledge of You." I was able to make it through without too many mistakes and was starting to feel the relief that comes from surviving traumatic experiences. Then one of the belly-dancing goddesses called to me from across the room, "You are some kind of attention hog, aren't you!"

As soon as she said it, my life passed before me. The room started to swirl, as a typhoon of shame began to suck me down the toilet of my soul. "Embarrassment" is an inadequate word when someone pins the tail on the jackass of what seems to be your most central core defect.

I am usually scrupulous about checking with people when I make requests for attention. But this time I was caught with my hand in the cookie jar up to the elbow. I remember slinking away in silent humiliation, putting my guitar back in its case and making a beeline for my car. I just wanted to get back to my lair to lick my wounds, and try to hold my self-hate demons at bay with a little help from my friend Jack Daniels. After that incident I quit playing music in public at all.

Several years later I was attending a very intense, emotional workshop with Dr. Marshall Rosenberg. Our group of about twenty people had been baring and healing our souls for several days. The atmosphere of trust, safety and connectedness had dissolved my defenses and left me with a innocent, childlike need to contribute. And then the words popped out of my mouth, "I'd like to share a song with you all." These words were followed by the thought: "Now I've gone and done it. When everyone turns on me and confirms that I have an incurable narcissistic personality disorder, it will be fifty years before I sing in public again."

Dr. Rosenberg responded in a cheerful, inviting voice. "Sure, go get your guitar!" he said, as though he were unaware that I was about to commit hara-kiri. The others in the group nodded agreement. I ran to my car to get my guitar, which I kept well hidden in the trunk. I was also hoping that I would not just jump in my car and leave. I brought the guitar in, sat down, and played my song. Sweating and relieved that I made it through the song, my first public performance in years, I felt relief as I packed my guitar in its case.

Then Dr. Rosenberg said, "And now I would like to hear from each group member how they felt about Kelly playing his song."

"Oh my God!" my inner jackals began to howl, "It was a setup! They made me expose my most vulnerable part and now they are going to crucify me, or maybe just take me out to the rock quarry for a well-deserved stoning!"

One by one, in a methodical clockwise direction, each person gave their individual reaction to my playing of the song. The first person said he was soothed by the melody, the second that she was inspired by the words. The third person said she had felt touched as it reminded her of someone precious that she loved. And on around it went, each person telling of a different need that was met, or another way he had been touched by my song. Dr. Rosenberg said he had felt inspired because I had mucked up the song a little in one place and had kept playing and finished it.

When everyone had shared, strong feelings began to pour into my body and up into my throat.

Gratitude and relief? No.

Joy? No.

Sorrow. Great sorrow, for all the years that I had not been playing. For all the people that could have been touched or inspired, had I given them the chance. For all the attention and connection I could have received but did not. As the sorrow eventually subsided like a passing rainstorm, warm powerful rays of sunny resolution began to radiate in my heart. It was a resolution and a clarity of commitment to myself to "perfect my selfishness." In a moment, I saw how playing the miserable martyr's role, sacrificing my passion to avoid disturbing other people, had too high a price. It also ripped other people off, by denying them what I had to give them. I swore then and there that I was not going to do that to me again.

I Don't Want To Do That To Me Again
by Ruth Bebermeyer

No use wasting life saying that I should have known better.
No use wasting time regretting what has been.
I just know I felt uneasy and I couldn't settle down,
Like my picture couldn't fit into that frame.
And I don't, don't want to do that to me again.

No use wishing now that I had not had to learn this way.
No use wasting time regretting what has been.
I just know I wasn't easy and I wasn't who I am,
But I guess I had to do it to see plain.
And I don't want to do that to me again.

I just want to go on singing the same tune I'm playing.
I want my self and my doing all the same.
And I want to walk in rhythm to the beat of my own soul.

When I'm out of step with me I'm into pain.
And I don't don't want to do that to me again.

The Treasure of Transparency

Recently I held a potluck dinner at my house for a group of friends, most of whom had been learning and practicing the techniques of Nonviolent Communication. After we had finished eating, a woman asked if the group would like to hear a story she wrote. At first no one answered, but then a couple of people asked how long the story was and whether the essence of it could just be told to them. Finally an agreement was reached about how the gift of the story could be given so that the group's needs for connecting with each other and relaxing at the party could also be met.

I was struck by how rare it is in this culture for individuals to be open and straightforward about their needs for attention in a social setting. It is equally rare for members of a group in American culture to honestly and openly express needs that might be in conflict with that individual's needs. This value of not just honestly but also openly revealing the true feelings and needs present in the group is vital for its members to feel emotional safety. It is also vital for keeping the group energy up and for giving feedback that allows its members to know themselves and where they stand in relation to others. These factors are important contributors to spiritual/psychological growth.

Usually group members will simply not object to an individual's request to take the floor — but then act out in a passive-aggressive manner, by making noise or jokes, or looking at their watches. Sometimes they will take the even more violent and insidious action of going brain-dead while pasting a jack-o'-lantern smile on their faces. Often when someone asks to read something or play a song in a social setting, the response is a polite, lifeless, "That would be nice." In this case, N.I.C.E. means "No Integrity or Congruence Expressed" or "Not Into Communicating Emotion." So while the sharer is exposing his or her vulnerable creation, others are talking, whispering to each other, or sitting looking as if they are waiting for the dental assistant to tell them to come on back. No wonder it's so scary to ask for people's attention.

In "nice" cultures, you are probably not going to get a straight, open answer. People let themselves be oppressed by someone's request—and then blame that someone for not being psychic enough to know that "Yes" meant "No."

When were we ever taught to negotiate our needs in relation to a group of people? In a classroom? Never! The teacher is expected to take all the responsibility for controlling who gets heard, about what, and for how long. There is no real opportunity to learn how to non-violently negotiate for the floor. The only way I was able to pirate away a little of the group's attention in the school I attended was through adolescent antics like making myself fart to get a few giggles, or asking the teacher questions like, "Why do they call them hemorrhoids and not asteroids?" or "If a number two pencil is so popular, why is it still number two," or "What is another word for thesaurus?"

Some educational psychologists say that western culture schools are designed to socialize children into what is really a caste system disguised as a democracy. And in one sense, it is probably good preparation for the lack of true democratic dynamics in our culture's daily living. I can remember several bosses in my past reminding me "This is not a democracy, this is a job." I remember many experiences in social groups, church groups, and volunteer organizations in which the person with the loudest voice, most shaming language, or outstanding skills for guilting others, controlled the direction of the group. Other times the pain and chaos of the group discussion becomes so great that people start begging for a tyrant to take charge. Many times people become so frustrated, confused and anxious that they would prefer the order that oppression brings to the struggle that goes on in groups without "democracy skills." I have much different experiences in groups I work with in Europe and in certain intentional communities such as the Lost Valley Educational Center in Eugene, Oregon, where the majority of people have learned "democracy skills." I can not remember one job, school, church group, volunteer organization or town meeting in mainstream America where "democracy skills" were taught or practiced.

Negotiating Needs From a Group

Many of us live much of our lives engaged, in various ways, with all sorts of groups: families, work groups, organizations, churches and social settings. We need to develop skills for negotiating our needs in relation to such groups. Because we were never taught how to powerfully and non-violently assert and negotiate our needs in a group, many of us either become resentful, suppressed sheep, or raging bulls running roughshod over others. We either "bowl over" or "roll over" in relation to others. We "bowl over" others out of the fear that we will not otherwise get what we want. Or we "roll over" out of hopelessness, feeling that we will never be able to get what we need.

It can be scary to ask for attention from a group because so often the group members are afraid to express their true feelings about your request. And most of us understand that when true negative feelings are withheld there will be some sort of consequence. In a group, the consequence is frequently shunning. (In every case of school shootings of which I am aware, the perpetrator was being shunned by most of the other students.)

Here are some tips to help you negotiate in groups:

1.   Practice presenting your requests for attention from a group confidently, so others can sense you will not be crushed if there is an objection.

2.   If you are scared when you are asking the group for something, be sure to say so. If you do not, it may be perceived as aggressive, because unexpressed fear often gets perceived as aggression.

3.   Be sure to give others time and space to check within themselves how they really feel about your request.

4.   Be ready to empathize with whatever the objection is. Don't get hung up on the content of their response. Instead, hear the feelings and needs behind the content. For example:

You: "I would like to share a story. Is that okay with everyone?"

Group Member: "No."

You: "Is that because you would like reassurance that it would take less than five minutes?"

Group Member: "No, it is because we have not made the decision yet about when our next meeting will be."

You: "Thanks for telling me. I would be happy to wait until after that decision is made. Would that work for everyone?"

5.   As in the example, after empathizing with the group member's response be prepared to check back within yourself to see if you have shifted. Have you changed your mind about what you requested? If not, either stay with the dialogue, or allow a solution to emerge that meets both your needs and the group's needs. Notice that in the example, the solution suggested is synergistic and would meet both your need to tell the story and the group member's need for the meeting time decision to be made.

6.   Be careful not to give in or give up after empathizing with the other's objection. If you do give "in" or "up" on what you want, you will resent the group for seeming to oppress you, and you will likely withdraw your participation. Or you will start gossiping about those that objected to your request and begin to build a splinter faction group that will weaken and sometimes even destroy the group. It is often the "nice" people who are so scared of conflict that do the gossiping that tears the group apart.

There can also be a particular problem with couples in a group. Sometimes a couple will form a faction splinter group. Then if they are upset about something going on in the group, they will collapse into collusion and gossip with each other, instead of airing their concerns with the whole group. Other times the factions are created along political lines or gender lines. With gender lines, frequently the men think the women are "too sensitive" and controlling. The women think the men are "too insensitive" and domineering. When these judgments are shared by people without Nonviolent Communication skills, they most often create painful unresolved conflict. When they are thought and not shared, it creates a tense depressed feeling in the group.

7.   Remember that after you have shared something of yourself in front of a group, you almost always need some kind of honest feedback in response. If you don't ask for this feedback, your mind will often project, onto the blank screen, nightmarish self-judgments which will serve to shut you down in the future. Example: You have just shared with the Committee to Create an Alternative School that you are afraid that the school will not be created in time for your five year old to attend and you will have to enroll her in public schools. You find yourself crying as you explain how important it is for you to protect her from the many kinds of violence found in public schools. Having cried, you feel vulnerable. You might ask: "I feel a bit vulnerable, having cried in public. I would like to know how people are feeling about what I have shared."

Then be prepared to empathize with the worst. Take a moment now to write down the three things that would be the most scary to hear after you have made yourself vulnerable and then asked for feedback. Here is what I came up with when I asked myself what would be scary feedback to receive and some possible empathic responses.

So I have cried in front of the Committee to Create an Alternative School and asked for feedback and heard back:

a.   From one of the other parents: "Don't try to manipulate us with those phony crocodile tears!" My response (hopefully): "So you don't trust my sincerity?"

b.   From a big burly man: "Oh God, give it up!" My response: "Sounds like you are disgusted with the show of emotion and would prefer we all discuss this practically and logically?"

c.   From a psychologist in the group: "You are just a little out of control, aren't you?" My response: "Are you concerned about straying from the agenda for the meeting? The psychologist's response to the above: "Yes, you are monopolizing the meeting." My response: "So you would like others to get equal time to speak? Yes, I am willing to give up the floor now." (Or, "I would like to make two more points if that's okay with the group.")

Ways to Feed Your Attention Hog

Honoring and owning your Attention Hog is a learned habit and skill. It must become a conscious and willful act in order to counter the cultural training we have received to pretend we do not want the attention. You will also be honoring others' needs to have their attention and appreciation received fully and gracefully.

1. When you are talking with someone and there is a radio or TV playing in the background, ask that it be turned off and not just down.

2. Ask groups to hear you play a new song you have learned.

3. Ask groups to listen to you read or recite poetry or prose.

4. Ask to be on TV or radio.

5. Submit articles for publication in magazines, newspapers or e-zines.

6. When speaking to a group, and people are talking in the background, say "My attention hog would like everyone's attention please."

7. When you are not getting the eye contact you would like from someone, ask for it.

8. If you want someone to call you more often, tell them specifically how often you would like to be called.

9. If you are not getting the recognition you want at work, ask your boss to write down a number of things that he sees you contributing to the business.

10. When receiving the applause of a group, take it in. Stand there looking at them until the entire wave of appreciation has passed.

Chapter

FILLING THE HOLE IN THE SOUL

I used to think that the need for approval was a misunderstood need for appreciation. In other words, the need for approval is the need for feedback that we are contributing to someone's well-being. But now I think we just need honest feedback about how we are affecting the life around us, for better or worse. This information can help us to make an informed choice about what we want to do about it and how to live our lives. This helps in the process of graduating from seeking others' approval, to meeting needs. We can then choose to meet others' needs when it fits for us, and our own needs when it does not.

One way we get approval is by shutting down or hiding our own needs. I remember being proud when the aunt who raised me would tell other people, "He's such a good boy" (this was before I hit my teen years). "He's such a good boy" meant that I was able to suppress almost all my needs, and never ask for anything. Of course, this had a cost. I developed tremendous resentment, which I acted out by stealing money from my aunt, and eventually running away from home, permanently.

A fun question I like to ask people is, "Do you want to be real or resentful? Are you willing to be honest about your needs or do you prefer to ignore your needs and take the resulting frustration out on yourself and others in destructive ways?" Your body and being will choose one or the other, consciously or unconsciously.

What's Your Default Setting?

Many people think by default. Instead of trying to get clear for themselves what their values are, they default to whatever their ministers, husbands, wives, or parents think. One problem with this kind of thinking is that it never leads to much satisfaction. Sure it fulfills other peoples' agendas, but never the individual soul's agenda for a fully lived life. It leaves us with that "hole in the soul" feeling that many of us spend a lifetime trying to fill, with addictions and achievements.

Another kind of *default* thinking is this: when anything goes wrong, or any time you are not happy, you start thinking about who's at fault. For example, if you are bored with your life, your *default* setting kicks in and you think: "God, my wife is boring, maybe I need a new one." Or the computer starts to go on the blink and you ask, "Honey, have you been messing with the computer?" Someone always has to be at blame when your inner computer has been programmed with a *default* setting.

Milk Every Compliment

If what we truly need is feedback, not approval, then what do we do when others compliment us? Compliments are one of the great joys in life and an important way of learning about how we are affecting others. Too often jackal thoughts — like, "I do not deserve this compliment," or "They must be trying to get something from me," or "Oh, my God! How do I respond to this?" — block us from receiving the energy and knowledge that would increase our sense of self-worth. It also prevents the giver of the compliment from having the joy of having their gift received. We can instead train ourselves to honor, celebrate and enjoy compliments.

When someone says to me, "Great workshop!" I almost always ask "Wonderful! What did you like about it?" Then I try to milk out these three things. One, I try to find out specifically what I said or did that they are reacting to. One lady said that I probed quickly to the heart of the pain that each person brought to work on. Two, I then asked her what needs of hers did that meet. She told me that during the course of her work with me, she had finally been able to see the humanness behind some of her son's actions, and that had given her hope for their relationship. Three, I then asked her for what feelings she was having about all this and guessing she felt "relieved." She said, "Relieved and hopeful for a better relationship."

When we had finished, I felt a deep sense of relief, and confidence that I truly had contributed to life. I was very glad that I had not just said "Thanks for the compliment." I am grateful I took the time to take it in, and empathize with the gratitude I was being offered. When I have talked to people later about how they felt about how I "took in" their compliment, I frequently hear things like, "I felt honored that you would take the time to receive my gift." Or, "I felt really heard, and that my compliment was genuinely appreciated." When someone gives you a gift package and you take the time to open it and pull out the shirt and put it on, it is a great gift back to the giver.

Chapter

THE DUTY GIVER

When people give something out of duty or guilt, they often become very demanding of appreciation for what they did, because they are getting no appreciation from themselves. In fact, often unconsciously, they feel resentful for what they did. This is what prevents them from taking in the appreciation from others even if it is offered. Often the appreciation is not offered because the request for it, spoken or unspoken, is perceived by the recipient to be a demand. Others sense that the gift came from duty and not love. Receiving from someone who is giving out of obligation often leaves one feeling like a worthless burden.

I remember overhearing my aunt and uncle (who took in me and my siblings when our parents split up) complaining to each other that they had given up their retirement to raise us kids. I remember the pain, guilt and worthlessness I felt in response. I remember wanting to disappear, eat less, take up less room. We also had a ritual around the dinner table. It started with my uncle looking at my brother and me with furrowed brow, which meant "You better not forget!" What we were not allowed to forget, under threat of physical beatings, was to say, "Thank you, Aunt Willie, the dinner tasted good." My Uncle Jake would listen very carefully to make sure we did not use that most subtle form of rebellion, the sing-song tone of voice school children use when they have to say "Good morning, Mrs. Tyrant."

If appreciation is offered to the person who has given out of duty, the "duty giver" will often have anger and resentment triggered and say things like "Well, it's about time!" or "Is that it? Is that all the thanks I get?" Because the duty giver's giving has not been an expression of love. Love giving is free-will giving, whereas the duty giver has given to avoid guilt and shame. My aunt was fond of saying, "I give and give and give—and all I ever get is a kick in the teeth." Even if people have offered sincere appreciation to such a duty giver, she will not be able to take it in until her self-resentment has been transformed through empathy into sorrow. What the duty giver needs is empathy for the resentment of having sacrificed his or her life energy for another, empathy for abandoning himself or herself, and for the loss of that self. When these people grieve for what they have done to themselves, they can even be grateful that others did not reinforce this self-sacrificing behavior by expressing appreciation for it.

So the first thing I would like the duty giver to do is grieve the cost of giving out of a role expectation, or duty. Many middle-aged women I see in my psychotherapy practice have great resentment and sorrow about the years they spent cleaning up after their husbands, or doing all the family laun*dreary*, with very little appreciation in return. They first need empathy for their resentment and then for the self-abandonment. How sad that they were taught that they must do their duty in order to deserve love.

The second thing I would like to offer the duty giver is compassionate understanding for what made them abandon themselves to "give" in the first place. In other words, I'd like them to become conscious and develop a nonjudgmental understanding of the dynamics involved. People often try to buy another's love through giving. They may be afraid of being judged as selfish or irresponsible if they do not "do their duty." They may act from an unconscious conformity to "doing the right thing."

This unconscious tendency to conform by giving in and compromising has a couple of elements worth discussing. One is the training we all receive about not hurting others physically or emotionally. This training does not usually make clear the difference between impact and cause. Nor does our typical cultural training say much about what we are responsible for and what we are not, nor about the primacy of intent. When Little Johnny laughs at his mother's new hat, he is told how evil he is and how he caused his mother's tears and pain. What craziness we could save Little Johnny if we could explain that the impact his laughter had on his mother was to trigger hurt, and that the cause of her hurt was not what he did, but what she thought when she heard Johnny laugh. It was mom's interpretation that Johnny didn't care about her feelings (and he should!) that hurt her feelings. She could have chosen instead to enjoy Johnny's amusement.

And what a relief it would be if Johnny's intention were acknowledged. Perhaps his intention was just to express surprise at a hat that reminded him of a cartoon peacock. Now Johnny may choose next time not to laugh when he sees someone's new hat out of compassion for the impact that it may trigger, but not out of fear or shame, or the belief that it is his sweet laughter that causes pain in others.

The other element that contributes to a compromising conformity is the lack of training we have in both asserting our needs and in continuing to negotiate once we have asked for something we want. Many of us are afraid to ask for anything because of fear that we will "cause" the other pain; and then we will, in turn, have guilt and shame triggered. We are also afraid of what we will tell ourselves when the other says no. In this polite culture we may also fear people saying "Yes" but meaning "No." They go along with our request but hold resentment toward us, and one day they will make us pay. I made my aunt and uncle pay every day, by having to look at my long face, deal with my constant foot-dragging, and live with my cold shoulder.

In this polite culture, pretended agreement permeates all the areas of our lives. There are people who say they will show up for an appointment and then do not, make agreements and then mysteriously break them, and pretend to be listening, but are mentally checked out.

I am particularly sad about people being afraid to assert their needs in the arena of physical affection. Because we are so thoroughly trained to give up on our needs when someone feels sad or hurt, we are often afraid to begin expressing any form of affection. We are afraid of the guilt we will feel when we reach a limit and tell the other person "No" to some request to go further with physical intimacy. We are afraid to start any physical expression of caring unless we intend to fulfill our "obligation" to "go all the way." We often feel obligated to totally satisfy the other person if they get aroused in any way. So much loving nurturing is missed because of these duty-bound, guilt-created beliefs. So much isolation, loneliness, distance and skin hunger are suffered because we think we are responsible for the other's needs. This is a result of a fear-based, duty-driven culture. It is possible to develop our own little subcultures within our culture—with values based on individual respect and autonomy. The Human Awareness Institute headquartered in San Francisco has been profoundly successful at this.

This fear of being held responsible makes it scary to even start to respond to others' or even our own needs. The moment someone thinks that they have the power to psychologically hurt or cause someone else's feelings, they enter into an ego maze of control struggles. To the degree I believe I can hurt your feelings, I live in the fear of guilt. To the degree I guide my behavior based on the fear of feeling guilty, I will begin to build resentment. This is Level 2, Stage 3 in Piaget, Kohlberg and Gilligan's book *Moral Development*. They call this Good Boy/Nice Girl Orientation.

When I'm afraid of feeling guilty, I will also gradually lose touch with my ability to empathize with others (Stage 6 of moral development) and my ability to guide my behavior with true empathy for the impact my actions make on others. When you give from duty, other people do not feel gratitude, and they aren't inspired to want to give back. "She did not do it because she loved me," we tell ourselves, "but because she's my mother or wife." The duty giver thinks people should be appreciative, which of course makes it all the harder to give it. They also think it's the duty of the receiver to give back appreciation. I heard one of these spiritual songs that said, "Love is always giving." If I believed in evil I would say that this is a truly evil concept. It takes something as precious as love and perverts it into something out of alignment with natural principles. Anything that you always give to you'll eventually kill, whether it is a relationship, a project, or anything else. Do you know what the major cause of death in houseplants is? Over watering. Also anything that only gives out without receiving in, runs out, drys up, or depletes itself. If you want your relationship to wither up and die, try to be all-giving.

The Codependency of Microzoophobia

It is my invariable custom to put out birdseed each morning and then sit back in my reading chair and watch the birds eat. My chair is fairly close to the feeder and I am aware that any quick movement on my part will scare the birds away. After five or ten minutes the first bird comes, and I notice myself take a small gulp of air and gently hold it in with slightly pursed lips. It is my attempt to control any bodily movement, even the rise and fall of my breathing chest, so as to not scare away the tiny creature. Another bird lands and I feel more pressure to control any movement, any sign of life in me that might frighten away my new flighty friends. I want to scratch an itch on my nose but I dare not.

Then it hit me, "These birds are controlling me. They will not let me breathe or move. They have taken over my will." My overactive imagination transforms the sparrow into the image of a giant pterodactyl, pinning me to the ground with its huge talons wrapped around my chest, preventing me from breathing as it decides whether to carry me back to its lair (Did pterodactyls have lairs?) or to eat me right there. Finally in one last desperate heroic lunge, I leap to my feet and discharge my lungs with a roar of power as I throw off the sparrow demons. The two birds at the feeder quickly fly back to safe refuge in a nearby tree as I revel in my reclaimed freedom. I imagine that one of the birds says to the other "Wow! Does this guy have autonomy issues or what?"

Do I do this with all my relationships? Lure them in with some kind of nurturing, project onto them a monstrous need to control my very life energies, and then chase them away in a fear-filled fit of rebellion?

I am particularly helpless if a cute kitten falls asleep on my chest. It might as well be a thousand-pound adult lion. I can lay there for hours debating the relative importance of our respective needs.

Voice One: "You have things to do that are much more important than this kitten's need to sleep."

Voice Two: "Oh, so now you are more important than the kitten. Remember what Gandhi said about how you can tell a man's character by how he treats the least of creatures around him."

Voice One: "You are just procrastinating."

Voice Two: "But it's so cute I hate to wake it up."

That one always gets me. So I lie there until the developing cramps trigger muscle spasms which jar the kitten awake. And this is only one of the painful symptoms of my disease: microzoophobia. That's the fear that small animals are controlling you. Now seriously, what hope do I have for a real relationship with an adult *Homo Sapiens* when I can not even iron out my autonomy issues with kittens and birds?

Do the Right Thing

Sometimes men say to me, "What's wrong with people doing the right thing?" I say to them, "I have two questions for you:

1. Has sex with your wife ever become a 'should' for her? Does she submit because it's the right thing to do since she's your wife?

2. And how exciting was the sex?"

Never do anything for other life forms. Only do things for your self, for the joy of giving. That way any appreciation that comes back to you is icing. And I only want "icing appreciation," never that flat monotone "obligation appreciation" I used to give my Aunt Willie after every boring meal so that my Uncle Jake would not cancel our fishing trip or thrash me. By giving only when it comes from the satisfaction of contributing to someone's well being, you get paid up front, always a good move. This way you can protect yourself from ever getting into the "collection business," trying to collect some appreciation or payback from someone for something you have done for them. If you ever find yourself in the collection business, I recommend you cut your losses (maybe you could even deduct it on your taxes and call it a business loss). But drop the account, let go of whatever you think you are owed, and mark up that loss in the "Education and Training Expenses" column. Learn from your loss, let it educate you. Next time be very conscious ahead of time whether you are wanting something back for whatever you are giving and tell the person up front what you expect back. This way you show them the respect of giving them a choice about whether they receive your services, given your fee.

Chapter

CONFESSIONS OF A CLING-ON

If a man is walking in a forest and makes a statement, but there is no woman around to hear it, is he still wrong? Or if a woman is walking in the forest and asks for something, and there is no man around to hear her, is she still needy? These Zen koans capture some of the frustrations people have with the opposite gender.

And where is the dividing line between someone simply having a need, and someone being a needy person? Is it written in heaven somewhere what is too much need, too little need and just the right amount of need for a "normal person?" Ask pop radio psychologists Dr. Laura, or Sally Jessie Rafael, or any number of experts who claim to know for sure, and you'll get some very different answers.

And isn't it fun to see the new sophisticated ways our advanced culture is developing to make each other wrong? You better keep up with the latest technical terminology or you will be at the mercy of those who do. Whoever has read the most recent self-help book has the clear advantage. Example:

Man: "Get real, would you! Your Venusian codependency has got you trapped in your learned helpless victim act, and indulging in your empowerment phobia again."

Woman: "When you call me codependent, I feel (notice the political correctness of the feeling word) that you are simply projecting your own disowned, unintegrated, emotionally unavailable Martian counterdependency to protect your inner ADD two year old from ever having to grow up. So there!"

Speaking of diagnosis, remember the codependent. Worrying about codependency was like a virus that everyone had from about 1988 to 1994. Here's a prayer to commemorate the codependent:

The Codependent's Prayer
by Kelly Bryson

Our Authority, which art in others, self-abandonment be thy name.
Codependency comes when others' will is done,
At home, as it is in the workplace.
Give us this day our daily crumbs of love.
And give us a sense of indebtedness,
As we try to get others to feel indebted to us.
And lead us not into freedom, but deliver us from awareness.
For thine is the slavery and the weakness and the dependency,
For ever and ever. Amen.

Thank God for self-help books. No wonder the business is booming. It reminds me of junior high school, where everybody was afraid of the really cool kids because they knew the latest, most potent putdowns, and were not afraid to use them.

There must be a reason that one of the best-selling books in the history of the world is *Men Are From Mars, Women Are From Venus* by John Gray. Although this book really does have many profound insights, could it be that our culture is eager for a quick fix? What a relief it must be for some people to think "Oh, that's why we fight like cats and dogs; it's because he's from Mars and I'm from Venus." Can you imagine Calvin Consumer's excitement and relief to get the video on "The Secret to her Sexual Satisfaction" with Dr. Gray-Spot, a picture chart, a big pointer, and an X marking the spot. Could that "G" be for "giggle" rather than Dr. "Graffenberg?" Perhaps we are always looking for the secret, the gold mine, the G-spot because we are afraid of the real G-word: Growth—and the energy it requires of us.

I am worried that just becoming more educated or well-read is chopping at the leaves of ignorance but is not cutting at the roots. Take my own example: I used to be a lowly busboy at 12 East Restaurant in Florida. One Christmas Eve the manager fired me for eating on the job. As I slunk away, I muttered under my breath, "Scrooge!"

Years later, after obtaining a Masters Degree in Psychology and getting a California license to practice psychotherapy, I was fired by the clinical director of a psychiatric institute for being unorthodox. This time I knew just what to say. This time I was much more assertive and articulate. As I left I told the director "You obviously have a narcissistic pseudo-neurotic paranoia of anything that does not fit your myopic Procrustean paradigm."

Thank God for higher education. No wonder colleges are packed.

What if there was a language designed not to put down or control each other, but nurture and release each other to grow? What if you could develop a consciousness of expressing your feelings and needs fully and completely without having any intention of blaming, attacking, intimidating, begging, punishing, coercing or disrespecting the other person? What if there was a language that kept us focused in the present, and prevented us from speaking like moralistic mini-gods? There is: The name of one such language is Nonviolent Communication.

Marshall Rosenberg's Nonviolent Communication provides a wealth of simple principles and effective techniques to maintain a laser focus on the human heart and innocent child within the other person, even when they have lost contact with that part of themselves. You know how it is when you are hurt or scared: suddenly you become cold and critical, or aloof and analytical. Would it not be wonderful if someone could see through the mask, and warmly meet your need for understanding or reassurance?

What I am presenting are some tools for staying locked onto the other person's humanness, even when they have become "an alien monster."

Remember that episode of Star Trek where Captain Kirk was turned into a Klingon, and Bones was freaking out? (I felt sorry for Bones because I've had friends turn into Cling-ons too.) But then Spock, in his cool, Vulcan way, performed a mind meld to determine that James T. Kirk was trapped inside the alien form. And finally Scotty was able to put some dilithium crystals into his phaser and destroy the alien cloaking device, freeing the captain from his Klingon form.

Oh, how I wish that, in my youth or childhood, someone had known how to apply a little Nonviolent Communication to free me from my Cling-on consciousness and communication. Just to have someone see me as a being with human needs and feelings instead of as a needy Cling-on would have been water to my desperately thirsty soul. Because I didn't get that, it has taken me many years to get to the point where relationships are "flowers for my table instead of air for my lungs," as my friend, Dr. Rosenberg, likes to say.

As a freshman at the University of Florida, it would have been so helpful to have run into just one Nonviolent Communicating girl. So that when I (in my Woody Allen, "I would never belong to a club that would have me as a member" consciousness said: "You wouldn't want to dance with me, would you?" I might have received a life-giving Compassionate Comeback like: "I wonder if you're a little nervous and maybe needing some reassurance that I am okay with being asked to dance?"

Then even if she told me "no," I could have held onto some shred of human dignity. Just a little demonstrated empathy for my present human experience would help me from getting swallowed up by my own inner judgments, screaming that I am a wimp for being scared and a needy parasite for being so hungry for human connection.

I have thought of myself as both parasite and host at different times in different relationships. In one relationship I would be the parasitic, needy, begging-puppy-dog, desperate victim Cling-on. In the next I would be the righteous, irritated, Vulcan, aloof, sophisticated, space-needing, guilty, abandoning, adult dog. Both leave me lonely and empty.

I remember being on the phone to a girlfriend who had been telling me her troubles for some 20 minutes. I remember beginning to think "This is the neeeeeeeeediest woman God ever put on this earth!" What I didn't know at the time was that "needy" does not have an independent existence. Needy is an interrelational word. It describes what is going on *between two* people; not *within one* person. When I am thinking that someone else is needy, it is because I have needs of my own coming up that I want met. However I am too scared of conflict or guilt to be conscious of my real needs, so I cope with my fear by dissociating from my body and needs to go up to my head to hallucinate a hellish dialogue about what is wrong with the other person. In this case, I started analyzing how insensitive she was for not using her intuition to know that I was tired and then offering to get off the phone without my having to ask her.

How sad that our culture teaches us to think in terms of what is wrong with the other when they do not give us what we want. How sad that our culture is based on "Judgment Games." We ask questions like, "Who's right and who's wrong? Who gets rewarded and who gets punished? Who is in the In Crowd and who are the losers?" Some cultures, like the agricultural Hopis, teach "Compassion Games." They ask different questions: "Who needs what, to be nurtured and grow? How can I make life more wonderful for you? Here's how you can make life more wonderful for me." Would not it be wonderful if our culture taught us that all our needs are opportunities for others to fulfill their life purpose by giving to us?

At that moment on the phone, the truth was that I was tired and wanted to rest but was too scared to say so. I was scared because I knew how guilty I would feel when she interpreted my need to rest as a rejection of her. All she would have to say is "I stuck my neck out and asked you for little support and now I feel abandoned by you," and I would go straight to guilt hell. If I were to be really nonviolently transparent with her, I might have translated my judgment of her as "needy" in the following way: "I am afraid to say this because you might feel hurt and then I might slip into feeling guilty, but I am tired and want to get off the phone now. How would you feel about us talking another time?"

Do I only have two options? The first, to violently stuff my feelings and needs and end up resenting myself for giving in and the other person for oppressing me. The second, to tell the truth about what I am feeling and needing and watch the other person get so wounded that they withdraw from the relationship. Or they attack me with anger or a guilt trip and I end up getting defensive or defeated by the guilt. Yuck! What happened to the Yum! and the Yea! of relationships?

Help, Mr. Sulu, I am lost! Which way back to the Milky Way of Love?

From the book *Nonviolent Communication* by Dr. Marshall R. Rosenberg, here's a North Star for finding the heart of honesty within oneself; which is the first step on the starry trek back to love.

"When _____ happens, I feel _____

because I want _____ . Are you willing to _____ ?"

For example: "When you did not visit me, I felt sad, because I wanted company. Would you tell me if you're willing to get together tomorrow?"

This is one way of focusing my thinking and communicating my truth accurately. Notice that the grammar of the sentence allows for no judgment of the other and requires that the speaker take responsibility for his feelings and needs. He takes responsibility for his feelings by declaring that his feelings are being caused by the condition of his needs. He does not say that his feelings are caused by the other person, but rather that if his needs are met, good feelings are produced; if not, bad or uncomfortable feelings are the natural result. He says "When you didn't come over, I was sad because I was wanting some company, could we get together tomorrow?" Not "I am sad that you didn't come over." This second statement does not make clear what is causing the sadness. The sadness is caused by the unmet need for company, not because a particular person does not come over. Sometimes people do not come over and you're glad, because you were wanting to sleep or read.

Notice that the last part ("Would you tell me if you're willing to") focuses on what you want done, right at the moment, to nurture you and/or bring you into connection with the other. Some of the most frequent requests I make are "Would you tell me what you heard me say?" when I am in need of understanding, or "How do you feel about what I said?" when I need feedback about where the other is in relation to me, or "Would you be willing to knock on the door first next time?" when I am wanting an agreement.

If I can notice what I am feeling, (I am lonely) I can know what I need (companionship) and then I have a chance of getting my need met (because I can ask you to spend time with me). All successful relationship begins with inner awareness. "Know thyself," as the Delphic oracle proclaimed.

I Can't Be In Touch With You
by Ruth Bebermeyer

I can't be in touch with you when I'm not in touch with me.
I can't see you when I'm looking for myself.
So if I seem to pass you blind, please try to keep in mind,
It isn't you, it's me I cannot find.

And here's a map, again from Dr. Rosenberg's book *Nonviolent Communication*, which uses the essence of empathy to find and feel the heart of the other. This will help you keep locked onto their humanness when they are upset and forget to look for it within themselves:

"When you see (or remember, or hear) _____ did you feel _____ because you were wanting _____? And would you like me to _____?"

For example: "When you heard that I was not coming to visit, did you feel disappointed because you were wanting some company? And would you like me to tell you if I am willing to call you tomorrow?"

As soon as I turn my attention to what my partner is reacting to, feeling, needing and requesting, I am in a different world. Instead of being caught in the control of her Cling-on tractor beam, which is about to suck me into the Black Hole of her endless need, I am being invited into the Secret Garden of a beautiful wonderchild, to play, and to give and receive nurturing. As I develop my skill to listen to and from my heart (my feelings and needs) I no longer see women and men as needy Cling-ons or detached Vulcans; only as sweet, sentient beings offering to meet my needs or requesting that I meet theirs. And when there is choice, all needs are beautiful.

These two "maps" (the first, a guide for expressing to others with self-responsible, non-judgmental honesty; the second, a guide for listening to others with accurate, non-judgmental empathy) are very simple in form. And yet, applying them in daily interactions has been the most difficult thing I ever tried to master. One thing that can help with mastery is practicing after the fact. For any situation that leaves a feeling of dissatisfaction, try translating it, using these two guides (doing it on paper, or even just mentally). Notice any shift of energy. Doing this may seem to take a lot of time and effort at first, but it *will* get easier and will also become more accessible in the moment. It's worth it! I personally know many relationships that these two maps have healed and saved.

One note of caution: this model or communication technique is a very powerful tool that can produce enormous life-serving benefits when applied with a strong intention to be compassionate with oneself and others. The intention must always be to connect and never to correct oneself or others. As with any tradition, institution, or structure, it must never be made more important than the people it was created to serve. The spirit of compassion must always take precedence over any idea of spiritual correctness. So please do not make a dreary dangerous religion out of it. And use it only as long as you are having fun with it.

Chapter

DO YOU WANT TO BE RIGHT,
OR HAVE MEANINGFUL RELATIONSHIPS?

"Jackass!" she says like a champion dart thrower, throwing a bulls-eye. Then all in one motion, she turns on her heel and storms out of the room. Suddenly I feel like a hit-and-run victim. Shock waves of shame shoot through me as the mushroom cloud of my worthlessness rises inside of me.

My female friend had just announced, with irritation and volume, "I want to talk to you right now!" And I, wanting to practice some newly learned communication skills answered, "You know, that tone triggers a lot of fear for me so I want to just continue to lie here looking at the ceiling."

How could my sweet, childlike honesty trigger such a verbally vile response? I was still lying down on my bed looking up, so I decided to project the "inner critic show" going on in my head onto the ceiling. The first character on stage was my original coping mechanism, my Neurotic, who blames himself whenever there is conflict. "Look at you, you are pathetic. You cannot even be there for your friend in her hour of need. And you call yourself a teacher of Nonviolent Communication."

As I started to put the shattered pieces of my ego back together, the roar of righteous indignation rose in my belly. Enter the character of my Character Disorder, who has graduated to blaming others whenever there is conflict. "Who the hell does she think she is? I'm not putting up with this rude, verbally abusive, boundary-invading perpetrator behavior!" It was of some relief to have my inner critic focus on someone else for a moment. Then my education pays off as my Therapist Complex offers the final analysis, "She is obviously suffering from a pseudo-narcissistic personality disorder with paranoid borderline tendencies."

As I lay there reveling in the safety of my righteous rage, it occurred to me that I was totally caught up in defensiveness. "What am I defending myself from?" I asked myself. "What is so scary?" The answer I discovered is that what is scary is the idea that "I may be in the wrong!" And my Belief System (BS for short) says that if I am wrong, I am a worthless piece of dirt, and therefore I deserve to feel the excruciating pain of shame that comes with this thought. My BS also tells me I deserve to be shunned and isolated from the rest of humanity, including my loved ones.

No wonder people fight so fiercely to appear to be "right." I believe that the bankrupt strategy of striving to be always right is a way of trying to create a sense of safety, socially and psychologically. You might say this obsession with being right is a fear-based drive to protect us from appearing to be "wrong." In a culture based on punishments and rewards, it is scary to ever be wrong for fear of various forms of punishment, like shunning, withdrawal of love, physical attack like corporal punishment, withholding of rewards, and other kinds of sanctions. Every experience of being wrong becomes psychologically associated with all the pains of punishments past. Most people in a "right/wrong" culture like ours are ever vigilant to protect from being cast as one of the wrong, bad people who are to be avoided, attacked, excluded, punished, blamed, and generally made into the scapegoats for the culture. This atmosphere of fear snowballs as people learn to quickly find someone to blame, rather than taking responsibility for their actions and learning from them. (Nurses have told me thousands of horror stories about how this policy of "cover your rear" perpetuates the same mistakes and causes irreversible damage and death in hospitals.) In other cultures making mistakes or "being wrong" about something is seen as an opportunity for growing closer through forgiveness and for learning something more. Do you want to be right or have meaningful relationships? You cannot have both!

-§-
I may be the detonator but I am never the dynamite. I may be the trigger for another's pain but the cause is their unmet needs.
-§-

Every situation, every relationship and every group we associate ourselves with is an opportunity to create the cultural climate that we want. We can create a climate of compassion or one of fear, depending on what we do with our mistakes and our judgments of ourselves and others.

Because I wanted to create a climate of compassion in the microcosm of my couplehood, I hunted in my memory for the tools with which to accomplish this. I remembered what Dr. Marshall Rosenberg said: "All judgments are the tragic expressions of pain and unmet needs." Perhaps this might even apply to my oh so right, sophisticated, clinical judgments? So I started to look for the pain in my body. Oh, there it is! Outrage! And what is the universal human need underneath the outrage? The need for respect, gentleness and safety. What else is in there? — because I know that anger never comes alone. There is always hurt or fear or something under it. Now I can feel it: Devastating hurt. A need for reassurance that I am valued.

As I lay there giving myself empathy, (i.e. paying attention to, and feeling into, what my reaction was all about), I start to feel a relieving shift in my body. The shift came as I allowed my awareness of my feelings to lead me into a reconnection with the life force within me. As soon as I am fully in touch with my true need, like the need to feel valued, I immediately feel the beautiful strength of it. (This is much different than staying up in my head meditating on images of "lack" or hunger to feel valued. This only produces more fear and pain.) I began to wonder if my friend was experiencing the same thing — hurt, and the need for reassurance that she is valued. I know that if I had tried to play lifeguard earlier, attempting to save her from drowning in her distress, it would have been a double drowning. I know that the undertow of my own unconscious reactions from my unhealed past would have prevented me from really being present. I had been drowning and needed to get myself to shore first before trying to throw her a line. Or as a wise man from the Middle East once said, "Get the dust out of your eye first, so you can see clearly to help someone else do the same."

-§-
When I am in pain, I want to wait till I am clear about what I want back from you before I speak.
-§-

After giving myself empathy, I was moved by compassion to go to my friend and see if I could offer her the understanding that would restore our connection. I am glad that I waited until my desire to connect with her came from my need to understand and reconnect, instead of from fear of abandonment, or guilt about abandoning her. I am glad I remembered the first commandment of nurturing relationships: Me first and only. I waited until my giving came simply from my heart, without any fear, shame, or guilt. Once this shift happens, the energy I give from is the same joy and innocence a child has when it feeds bread to a hungry duck.

"When I heard you call me a jackass a while ago, were you feeling angry and hurt because you were needing reassurance that your need to be heard mattered?" Her eyes started to fill with tears and a faint outline of a smile started to creep across her lips as she said, "It's about time, Jackass."

"Yes, I'm guessing that was painful for you, and you would have liked this quality of listening earlier," I said. "Yes," she said, the tears now flowing freely. "But I am also relieved that you waited till you were really in a position to do so instead of trying to give me empathy from hell — and then resenting me."

How beautiful to finally see the truth behind her calling me "Jackass." How beautiful to finally hear that my dear friend is in pain and wanting some reassurance from me that she matters. This allows me to actually enjoy my partner's pain. I do not mean this in the sadistic sense. I mean that there is a distinct joy in the intimacy of feeling the same feeling with another even if it is some type of pain. There is also a sense of relief in the awareness that as I am present to my partner's pain, she is being assisted in going deeper into and therefore through her pain. As John Bradshaw says: "The quickest way out of pain is through it." I am glad I gave her my honesty, (i.e. that her tone of voice had triggered my fears, and that I wanted to lie there awhile) because it ultimately led to a deeper level of intimacy.

Stan Dale, founder of the Human Awareness Institute, defines the word "intimacy" as "into me you see." And my honesty gives those around me a window into my inner workings.

When a wound gets triggered in me by what someone says, I am not truly hearing what was said. What I heard was my own inner Character Disorder voice making them wrong, or my Neurotic making me wrong, or responsible for their pain. How sad that we take so much *responsibility for* our loved ones' pain. When we do, we are completely blocked from being *responsive to* the feelings or needs of the other. We can be reactive to the pain in the other and give them something out of fear, shame or guilt—but we cannot be empathetic to the other when we think we *should* or because we feel we *have to*. Also, giving is not a very joyful unless we are being responsive *to* the need of the other, instead of responsible *for* them. When I think I am responsible for the hurt of another, I am not really present. I am off on a guilt trip to Siberia in my head.

> -§-
> If I heard blame, I misunderstood your pain. If you heard blame, please try to hear my pain again.
> -§-

So in order to prevent myself from feeling guilty, or from seeing my partner as being "ugly," I remember that communication is always either an SOS or a care package. Then I imagine my partner singing me this song:

See Me Beautiful
By Red and Kathy Grammer

See me beautiful, look for the best in me.
That's what I really am and what I want to be.

> It may be hard to find, and it may take some time, but see me beautiful.
> See me beautiful, each and every day.
> Could you take a chance? Could you find a way?
> To see me shining through, in everything I do, and see me beautiful?

Sending Your Relationship an SOS

Here are some ways to save your relationship from fear, shame and guilt trips.

1.   PACK A Q-TIP. Quit Taking It Personally (again from Stan Dale). Below are some ways I have learned to Q-TIP.

a.   When I am listening to others, I want to listen with an awareness that their pain is coming from their unmet need—not from my behavior. People are never angry or upset with us; they are distressed about an unfulfilled need of their own. I may be the detonator but I am never the dynamite. I may be the trigger for their psychological pain, but I am never the cause. One way of training my consciousness to stay focused on this truth is to speak this truth either in my mind or out loud to my partner.

-§-
As soon as I jump to solution, I lose connection with the other's needs.
-§-

Suppose your partner says she is angry because you did not call her. Taking it personally while trying to give understanding, you might say, "Are you feeling hurt because I did not call you?" You are now taking responsibility for her pain. It is this thinking that punches your ticket to the jail inside yourself. Do not pass go, do not collect 200 kisses.

Here's the same statement using a Q-TIP: "Are you feeling upset because you were needing reassurance that you matter, and want me to agree to call you earlier next time?"

b.   Make sure you understand the universal human need being expressed by your partner instead of jumping to thoughts about solutions. Example: Your girlfriend tells you she is dissatisfied with the sex you're having. If you jump straight to a solution, you might say, "Well maybe you need to find somebody new." Instead, you can feel—sense, look into—what her need might be. Maybe she is needing some empathy for how scary it is to ask for what she wants in the bedroom.

c.   Remove your grandiose self from your partner's need. She never actually needs you to take the trash out. Her need is support; her request is that you take the trash out. She does not need you to go to the movie with her; she needs companionship and requests you to fill that need. Or perhaps if she were more honest she might say "I am needing some financial support. Would you be willing to take me to the movie?" If I do not keep this straight, I start to see my partner's needs as nooses around the neck of my autonomy and freedom. Or I see her needs as burdens I have to fill — or suffer the consequences of her withdrawal or my guilt.

One way I keep this in focus is by thinking or saying "Are you feeling overwhelmed because you are needing some help right now?" If I want to feel as though I have a ball and chain on my leg, I ask, "Are you feeling overwhelmed because you need *me* to help you?" Read those two sentences again and you will understand how, with a small difference in wording, you remove yourself as the solution to your partner's need. You don't have to take responsibility for the other person's need. You could just understand and empathize with it.

2.   CALL A TIME OUT. Just say "I'm _____" and then the truth about your present emotion. Like "I'm scared right now about the tension between us and I want to be alone for a while." Remember that — unlike basketball or other sports — you have unlimited time outs. Be sure you have a private place you can go to just be with your self. Bring your journal to write out what is going on inside you. Also bring your cell phone and your list of phone numbers for your support team. It gives me an incredible sense of security to have this rich resource of a team of "empathy exchange" part-

-§-
The right road has room for only one. Do you want to be right or have company?
-§-

ners. We take turns listening to each other when our stuff is up after being triggered. It is also one of the things that most helps me grow and keeps stability in my relationships.

If I am sensing that our argument is starting to tear at the fabric of our relationship, I like to remember that I am a member of the 4R Club (similar to the 4H Club). The privileges of this club allow me to enjoy the four Rs: Relax, Recharge, Replenish, and then Return to my beloved. When I return, I come from a higher, fear-less perspective, which allows me to have more empathy for my beloved and see a more productive direction for our discussion.

3.   CREATE AND USE A PASSWORD. Once my partner was in pain about our relationship and said "Any self respecting woman would leave you!" I jokingly responded, "Does that mean you're staying?" We laughed till we cried. After that, many a time when things got tense, we could just say, "Does that mean you're staying?" And the tension would dissolve into laughter.

Five Ways to Torpedo Your Relationship

Relationships based on being right are really not relationships at all. They are "relation-dinghies" (Stan Dale's word). That is because they are based on the fear of being wrong, which is an attitude and an energy that contracts and constricts life and relationships. But please do not make yourself wrong for being caught up in the fear of being

-§-
Relationship
Hell =
Being very
sensitive to
your part-
ner's pain
and taking
responsibili-
ty for it.
-§-

wrong. After all, you grew up in a culture which is constantly asking "Who is right, and who is wrong?" and "Who shall we reward, and who shall we punish?" or "Who shall we include and who shall we exclude?"

On the other hand, just because we grew up in that kind of a culture does not mean we need to keep creating it in our present relationship. I recommend we ask different questions, like "How could I make your life more wonderful?" and "Would you like to know how you could make my life more wonderful?" and "What are your needs right now?" and "Would you like to know what I need right now?" Now, if none of this appeals to you, here are some suggestions to help you prevent your relation-dinghy from growing into a relation-ship:

1.   Keep your attention focused at all times on who is right or wrong in a discussion, fair or unfair in a negotiation, selfish or unselfish in giving (it helps to keep a list of who has done what for whom), kind or cruel in their tone of voice, rude or polite in their man-

nerisms, sloppy or neat in their dress, and so on. Be careful not to realize that your attempt to be right is really an attempt to protect yourself from thinking you are wrong and then feeling shame.

2.   If you need some support for this, I recommend certain self-help groups who can give you the latest scoops on the most powerful, politically correct labels with which to overpower and confuse your partner. Members of these groups will collude with you in validating that your partner really is a man or woman who is commitment-phobic, emotionally unavailable, counterdependant, needy, spiritually unevolved, dysfunctional, immature, judgmental, sinful, bi-polar, OCD, clinically depressed, or experiencing adult-onset ADD. It is important to keep your consciousness filled with such terminology to prevent any fondness from developing. This also helps for keeping you caught in the "paralysis of analysis" and clueless about what you or your partner are needing from each other.

3.   Adopt this test for love: If your partner really loves you, he or she will always know what you want even before you know—and then give it to you without your having to go through the humiliation of actually asking for it. And your partner will do this regardless of the sacrifice it requires. If your partner does not give you what you want, choose to believe it means he or she does not love you.

4.   Ask for what you do not want instead of what you do want. I heard of a man who asked his wife to stop spending so much money shopping. She took up gambling on the internet.

5.   In case your relationdinghy starts to grow, here are a few torpedoes guaranteed to sink it again:

"It hurts me when you say that."

"I feel sad because you…fill in the blank (won't say 'I love you' or 'I'm sorry,' won't have sex, won't marry me, etc.)"

If you really want to choke the life out of any relationship, meditate on "I need you." Then you will know how I felt for about thirty-five years of my life. I felt like a drowning swimmer and I would grab hold of anyone who came near me and try to use them as a life raft. Now I truly prefer that relationships be flowers for my table instead of air for my lungs.

When I Come Gently To You
by Ruth Bebermeyer

When I come gently to you I want you to see
It's not to get myself from you, it's just to give you me.
I know that you can't give me me, no matter what you do.
All I ever want from you is you.
I know your fear of fences, your pain from prisons past.
I'm not the first to sense it and I'm plainly not the last.
The hawk within your heart's not bound to earth by fence of mine,
Unless you aren't aware that you can fly.
When I come gently to you I'd like you to know
I come not to trespass your space, I want to touch and grow.
When your space and my space meet, each is not less but more.
We make our space that wasn't space before.

Chapter

HEALING THE BLAME THAT BLINDS

Blame is the game that blinds me from understanding the true cause of all my emotional distress. When I am blaming, I am unaware that my anger, fear, shame and guilt come from the part of me I call "the inner critical voice" or, affectionately, my Inner Jackal. As long as I keep the big bony finger of blame pointed in your direction, I can remain unaware that it is the story I am telling myself about your behavior that is stimulating my painful reactions. This lack of awareness of the true cause of my distress also keeps me powerless to do much about it. And even though I may make great efforts to douse this distressing fire inside me by ensnaring you into taking responsibility for it, the fire still burns. It is as though there were a mirror reflecting a fire, and I continue to pour bucket after bucket of water on the mirror, expecting to put out the fire. Whenever I hold anyone as guilty, I disempower myself.

Another way to look at blame is, to use Dr. Rosenberg's phrase, as a tragic expression of an unmet need. When I call you "selfish," I am expressing my own disappointment. I want you to give more consideration to my needs. When I call you "stupid," I am usually expressing frustration about my wanting you to have been previously aware of certain information. When I call you a "jerk," I may be scared and wanting more space between my car bumper and yours.

Blame is an ineffective request for empathy, and for consideration of my unmet wants and inner pain. The tragic part is that the form I have chosen to express my request makes it difficult for others to give to me without harming the relationship. This is not only true of requests I make of others, but also those I make of myself. This morning I tried to motivate myself to get out of bed early and write this chapter by telling myself that I was lazy and self-sabotaging if I did not. Well, that was such an unpleasant nagging voice to hear so early that I rolled over and went back to sleep.

-§-
Only when your beloved trusts that her expression of either "no" or "yes" will maintain the same quality of connection between you both, can there be deep safety in the relationship.
-§-

So what can be done about this habit of making requests of ourselves and others in the form of blame? Just as blame is a protective move based on fear and ignorance, compassion is a corrective countermove based on courage and understanding. Whenever I find myself blaming myself or others, I turn my attention to that part of my body from which the feeling of blame originates. Sometimes it is in my stomach, and I know from experience that this is the location of my anger. Sometimes it is my heart area, and I know I'm feeling hurt. If it is my upper chest, that means fear. It is a relief to acknowledge it, feel into it and imagine what it wants in order to feel better. Now I am ready to try what Marshall Rosenberg calls "Giraffe Speak." Now I am ready to take responsibility for what I am wanting, and for what I am feeling. I am willing now to "stick out my long neck" and reveal my true feeling of the moment and ask for exactly what I want.

Now, instead of calling you inconsiderate, I might say "I feel lonely and want you to come over." Instead of calling myself lazy, I might tell me, "I am feeling scared and want you to finish this chapter before the deadline." Giraffe Speak is not a technique to manipulate, but a way of increasing your chances of inspiring compassion and cooperation from yourself and others.

The reason blame is so rampant is that it seems like it works. A mother tells her grown son that he is ungrateful because he does not phone often enough. So the son starts calling weekly. Did the mother get what she wanted? Maybe on the surface, but not without harming the relationship. Yes, the son is calling, but only because he feels too guilty, ashamed, or scared not to. And the deeper longing the mother has for connection with her son will continue to be unmet. How painful for her to hear her son's flat monotone voice saying, "Hi, Mom, here's your weekly call."

Another popular feature of blame is its usefulness in extracting sweet revenge on our hated ones. Aside from my private practice, I work with gang kids and their families in Southeast San Diego. I have noticed that few things seem to delight the kids more than to catch one of the counselors breaking the rules and then to point their own big bony finger of blame at them. When you ask the kids why this brings them such joy they say, "Cause now they know how I feel all the time when they yell at me for stuff." Again I can see how this blaming and trying to get revenge is a poorly coded SOS for understanding and empathy. Sadly, blaming is hereditary, in the sense that English or French are hereditary. Just as you inherit your native language from your parents, so too do you inherit the cultural patterning of using blame to coercively get your needs met. It is also contagious and addictive.

-§-
What makes me not free is my fear of abandonment or loss.
-§-

Self-blame is the same game. It is an attempt to get some relief, through revenge, on ourselves. And again this self-blame is a poorly coded SOS for help in the form of self-understanding, empathy and compassion. I have tried to affirm the self-critical voices away, only to create more polarization.

The Voice: "How could you be so stupid?"

Me: "I am a perfectly intelligent person."

The Voice: "How could anyone like you?"

Me: "I am a perfectly lovable person."

The dialog goes on and on. Inside of us the crying gets louder, like an ignored child, or takes another form in an attempt to get heard. Sometimes it takes the form of self-sabotage, relationship or work addictions, spiritual addictions, or depression.

I want to maintain a clear intention of compassionately connecting with the feelings and needs underneath any blame I hear, whether inside or outside of me. As long as I am sweetly connecting to the feelings and needs, I am feeling wonderfully alive. However, many times I get to a place of feeling overwhelmed, and that is when I reach out to someone in my community for understanding. If I happen to ask you for understanding, please remember not to try to solve my pain with New Age chicken soup, like, "Why have you created this in your life?" or "Well, I am sure it is all part of the universe's perfect plan for your life," or "You'll probably need to increase your zinc and calcium intake." There's also conventional chicken soup, like "Things could be worse," and "No pain, no gain."

-§-
"There is luxury in self-blame. When we blame ourselves we feel no one else has the right to."
—Oscar Wilde
-§-

Words are Windows or They're Walls
by Ruth Bebermeyer

I feel so sentenced by your words, I feel so judged and sent away.
Before I go I've got to know, is that what you meant to say?
Before I rise to my defense, Before I speak in hurt or fear,
Before I build that wall of words, tell me did I really hear?

Words are windows or they're walls
They sentence us or set us free.
When I speak and when I hear
Let the love light shine through me.

There are things I need to say, things that mean so much to me.
If my words don't make me clear, will you help me to be free?
If I seemed to put you down, if you felt I didn't care,
Try to listen through my words to the feelings that we share.

> Words are windows or they're walls
> They sentence us or set us free.
> When I speak and when I hear
> Let the love light shine through me.

Judgement Slows Growth

Psychological judgments and diagnoses often trigger hopelessness because they are static. By "static" I mean words that label what we "are" — as in, "You *are* paranoid" or "You *are* immature." These kinds of labels offer no room for change, development or growth, but by virtue of their static nature perpetuate the status quo. So instead of even thinking that someone is a paranoid, I prefer to think "I am sad about how often this person says he is afraid." Or instead of thinking that someone is immature, I would prefer to think "This person is growing more slowly than I would like" or "They are at a certain level of development."

Everything can be expressed in terms of my reality instead of your abnormality. Instead of saying you are "commitment-phobic," I could say I am frustrated with how long it is taking you to make certain agreements.

Sometimes our judgments of others lead us to punish them by withdrawing our love. Withdrawing love from a child usually inspires self-recrimination in that child. This is why most of us, myself included, are so harsh on ourselves. What is really needed is continued presence and acceptance by the parent, so that security can be felt by the child. Once the child feels secure and free of anxiety, she can empathize, turning her attention toward the feelings of others.

If the child does something like hit someone and the parental response is to yell at the child, that parent is interfering with the child's moral development. The yelling parent will trigger fear in the child, which shuts down the child's emotional body, including her sense of empathy for the person she is hitting. Even if the child "learns not to hit" others, her motivation for not hitting others is based on a fear of punishment, which is a much lower level of moral development than compassion for others. And besides, frequently what is learned is simply, "Don't hit little brother when Mom or Dad are watching." Nothing bad happens when Mom and Dad are not watching so it must be okay to hit him then.

If the parents are present to the child, this supports the child in turning her attention toward how other people feel. This is the beginning of empathy for other people, which developmentally is the most mature form of morality. This helps the child evolve beyond the self-absorbed stage of trying to avoid punishment or gain rewards. It supports the child in developing a holistic, ecological relationship with his social environment. Self-recrimination slows down discrimination. As one ruminates on what one should have done or what one is (lazy, stupid, mean, needy) for having done some action, no thought goes into noticing the choices one made that created the undesirable outcome.

-§-
The impulse to attack comes from the fear of being attacked. The impulse to blame comes from the fear of being blamed.
-§-

Our mind is absorbed with the fear, shame and guilt that self-judgmental thinking creates. No thought goes into what choices could have been made to create a different outcome. No thought goes into understanding what made the person make the those undesirable choices in the first place. No thought goes into how to gather the resources and skills to make different choices, take different actions and therefore create different outcomes. We are thinking we "should have known better" instead of thinking about how we could "know better in the future."

We have been taught to withdraw our own self-acceptance when we do something that creates an undesirable outcome. This withdrawal of self-acceptance undermines the secure base from which we might critically, or maybe I should say uncritically, examine our choice and thinking processes. To put it crudely, we have been taught to think in a way that keeps us stupid (i.e. keeps us from learning as quickly as we might). Perhaps even more tragically, it contributes to a sense of harsh self-doubt. This self-recriminating thinking contributes to a lessening of self-caring and self-respect. It is a good way to prevent us from knowing better in the future. Self-respect, that most precious of all experiences, is lost in a labyrinth of self-recriminating analysis.

Re-Viewing Victimhood

There has never been a perpetrator that did not first see himself as a victim. Feeling victimized is the precursor to perpetration.

There certainly are people who have been raped, beaten, stolen from, and so on. But those people still have a choice about whether they think of themselves as victims. It is only by thinking of oneself as a victim that certain perpetrator dynamics are set in motion. Of course it is extremely difficult when one has been physically injured, for example, not to look at the event through our victim culture's glasses. When we have grown up in a society where everyone completely agrees that the earth is flat, all laws and ideas of justice are based on that assumption. In such a society it is practically impossible to hold a "world as round" perspective.

Our flat earth society believes that everything can be understood in black or white, either/or, victim or perpetrator, good or bad terms. The answer to all problems, and the definition of justice, is to reward good behavior and punish bad behavior. This too is the conclusion of the John Wayne think tank on sociopolitical policy. Because it is obvious who the good guys are, since they wear white hats and all the bad guys wear black hats (or turbans), any fool can administer justice. Just like big John, we can buy drinks for all the good guys. And as for the bad guys? Shoot them!

What will it take for us to transform our victim/perpetrator, good guy/bad guy, Wild West mentality into something less adversarial? It requires leaving the safe shores of our society's—and our loved ones's—worldview, and venturing into the uncharted waters of our own examined experience. We must go beyond the comforting sympathy of those who would collude with us in our powerlessness and choicelessness.

I once had a workshop participant say to me, in a provocative tone of voice, "What choices would you have if someone were torturing you baby daughter right in front of you?"

"I would have two choices," I answered. "One would be to have compassion for my daughter and her torturer and for the pain in my own heart watching, and the second would be to express my own pain, passionately and nonviolently." I answered.

"No," said my questioner, "You would have no choice but to be enraged and wounded by what was happening."

"No," I said. "I would have another choice, although I agree that from the common worldview you would have only one choice. But remember Jesus's words hanging from the cross, 'Father forgive them, for they know not what they do.'"

Responsibility for Choice = Power

If I let you accidentally oppress me, use me, or take advantage of me, I need to apologize to you as a way of reclaiming my power. I want you to know I regret developing the resentment that always comes when I abandon speaking up for myself, and allowing you to get your needs met at my expense.

-§-
Blaming or harming another person is a strategy to get relief from our feelings of powerlessness and hurt.
-§-

Under a section entitled "Putting Aside the Blame," in the book *Difficult Conversations*, Stone, Patton and Heen of the Harvard Negotiation Project Group write, "When you learn of your wife's infidelity, you want to say, 'You are responsible for ruining our marriage! How could you do something so stupid and hurtful?!' Here, you are focusing on blame as a proxy for your feelings. Speak... more directly about your strong feelings—'I feel devastated by what you did.'"

How sad that even here, where we are being coached by some of the brightest minds in the U.S., we are taught to not take any responsibility for our own reactions. Instead, we are instructed to hold the other person responsible. "I feel devastated by what you did," suggests that it is what the other person did that directly caused the reaction, implying that there is no space between cause and effect. And of course believing that you have no control over your reaction to someone else's behavior leaves you feeling powerless. As Rollo May points out in his book *Power and Innocence,* powerlessness is the precursor to violence. The Watts riots in the 60s demonstrated this. The feeling of powerlessness also makes it easier to deny any choice about how one expresses the pain or anger that was triggered by the other. After all, it is commonly thought, the other person caused you to be overwhelmed and devastated, which caused you to go out of control.

The feeling of powerlessness also frequently leads to the strategy of trying to control the stimulus. And when you can't control the stimulus, this can trigger an overwhelming sense of inadequacy — which can lead to trying to destroy the stimulus, like O. J. Simpson (assuming he did the killing). Domestic violence stimulated by perceived infidelity is a leading cause of death among women.

I never want to think that the other person has the power to determine my reaction. They do not, unless I think they do and thereby let them. So instead of saying or even thinking, "I am devastated that you secretly had sex with another man," I would rather say, "When I found out that you had sex with another man, I felt deeply sad and angry. I felt a great loss of trust. I need openness, communication, and to be trusted with the full truth. Can you explore what needs you were trying to meet by making this choice and not telling me?" By thinking and speaking this way, I empower myself with the understanding that I have a choice about how I respond. I acknowledge that my pain is not caused by the other but by my unmet needs. And I have choices about how and where to get my needs met.

-§-
When I am judging, I am trying to hold someone else responsible for what I am feeling.
-§-

Chapter

FROM FIGHTING FAIR TO FUN FIGHTING

Have you ever heard the term "fighting fair?" Self-help guru John Bradshaw uses the term to describe a set of principles he uses to teach conflict resolution between couples. However, I think "fighting fair" is an argumentative term in itself. Since when has anybody ever agreed on what "fair" is? If we agreed on that, we would not be fighting in the first place. It starts you off on a right v. wrong adversarial footing. The idea sends you up to your head to be ever vigilant, like a lawyer ready to pounce. "Objection, Your Honor, 'fair' is not truly an objective term, because it puts the authority in some subjective external body." And if our lawmakers, judges, clergy, psychologists, gurus and philosophers cannot agree on what "fair" is, what chance do we common folk have?

I prefer a much more subjective reference: "Fun Fighting." The locus or center of this authority is within me. "Am I having fun yet?" This helps me take the responsibility for whether I am having fun and if not, what I am going to do about it. By fun I do not mean just the pleasure of amusement; I mean the satisfaction of being in genuine connection with someone and moving the dialogue forward.

Thinking for one second that something is not "fair" is poison to potent, productive problem-solving. When I think something is not fair, my consciousness is focused on an image of myself as powerless victim. When I hold that image of myself as a victim of some powerful unfair force, very few of my brain cells are working on the problem at hand. My feelings are a mix of anger, hurt and hopelessness. I have very little awareness of my present need; therefore, I have little hope of taking an action that might meet that need. I would prefer to notice that I am confused about how to get my needs met in that moment. I

-§-
When someone is upset with you, keep focusing on what their needs might be, instead of thinking about what is wrong with you.
-§-

would like to step back from the particular strategy that I am locked into (like persuading my partner that buying her a new car right now would not be fair to me), and get more connected and conscious of the underlying need. The need might be to reassure myself that I will take good care of my resources, or that I will negotiate powerfully and nonviolently for my own interests. From this perspective, I might find a way to embrace her needs also and look for a win/win solution. Often it is being locked into my judgment of the other as unfair that traps me into tunnel vision of one solution.

Because this singlemindedness of purpose shows no interest or empathy for the needs of others, it usually triggers rebellion. If the other submits, there will be foot-dragging, broken agreements, passive-aggressive sabotage or some form of payback. With rebellion comes fear and resistance in the other person, who digs in to protect her interests. No one likes to submit to another person out of fear of their judgment. No one likes to think they are losing in any interaction.

When Push Comes To Hug

Relationships are like Chinese finger puzzles. You know the kind made of straw, where you scrunch up the cylinder and put both your index fingers in each end. If you try to pull your fingers back out again, the cylinder tightens, and holds your captive fingers all the tighter. The key to getting out of the Chinese finger puzzle is the same key as getting out of the polarized power struggle in a loving relationship. It is useful to push toward the middle instead of pulling toward your own ends. When you find yourself struggling toward one of the polar ends of an apparent conflict of needs, the strain of the power struggle can be decreased by pushing back toward the middle, as counter intuitive as this is. As furiously as I might try to get my point across or have my needs heard, if I use the same amount of energy to show understanding for the other's position, I will ease the power struggle and move us toward resolution. I choose to fight toward the life, toward the connection with each other, which is the common life-force that sustains and connects us. This helps protect us from getting caught up in a fight to the death.

One form this life energy takes is our needs. Because we all have the same needs for connection, freedom, celebration, physical sustenance, inspiration, peace, and so on, expressing our needs clearly to each other is a powerful way to get us connected and giving to each other.

Some of the central apparent conflicting needs in intimate relationships are: freedom v. closeness, traditional marriage v. open marriage, autonomy v. interdependence, aliveness v. security. Maybe there is a law of the universe that make opposites attract. It makes all the spendthrifts find the misers, the slobs find the anal neatniks, the intellectuals find the emotionals, the extroverts find the introverts, the action-oriented find the being-oriented, the harmony-seeking find the adventurous, those seeking certainty find those wanting spontaneity, and so on. It is true

-§-
If you want to keep the wild in your wild man, keep encouraging him to keep setting himself free.
-§-

with any tug-of-war, that as soon as you move toward the other's position, all the tension goes out of the struggle, and it can turn into a hug of love.

I want to push toward my partner. I want to push in toward intimacy instead of just pulling out toward my desired outcome. So when my partner is pulling for closeness and I find myself tugging back for freedom, I can change the polarity of the conversation by just beginning to think: "How can I meet some of her needs for closeness without compromising my needs for freedom?" As soon as I start thinking this way, the field of energy between us will begin to soften and relax. The tension will decrease. The fear that we have to fight, defend and protect ourselves to get our needs met will diminish in both of us.

How To Have a Fight To the Life

When blaming is going on, which is another way of saying that a request for empathy, healing and reconnection is being made, I recommend taking one of the actions listed below. The order of these actions is hierarchical from most effective to least. I need also to be humble enough to recognize which of these actions I can do with honesty and integrity. By humble I mean that I am not overestimating my level of skill or present state of mind. I need to hold an accurate assessment of my ability to be present, and not be thinking I "should" be empathic, compassionate or more present than I am. For example, even if I recognize that empathy would probably be the most effective strategy for the occasion, I will still need to choose honesty at that moment if that is all I can give with congruence.

A simple guideline is: Give empathy when you can, and honesty when you can't. For example, imagine your partner saying, "You just are not meeting my needs for relationship. And besides that you are selfish." Here are some of the ways you could respond:

1. Empathize with the pain and unmet needs, of which the blame is a tragic expression. You might say: "Are you feeling kinda lonely and hurt, and need more consideration of your needs?"

2. Express any regret you have for anything you've done—or haven't done—that might have triggered your partner's pain. (Remember, you could not possibly cause it, only trigger it.) You might say: "I am sad that I forgot your birthday and went to play golf all day because I would have liked to have been there for you when you needed support."

3. Ask your partner for acknowledgment. You might say: "I am sad and would appreciate acknowledgment that I did remember your birthday for the last 6 years."

4.   Ask your partner to acknowledge her regrets or actions. You might say: "I am frustrated and would appreciate acknowledgment that you forgot my birthday too, and I would like to hear how you felt about forgetting."

5.   Give nonviolent self-responsible honesty. You might say: "I am feeling scared right now and need to protect myself from sinking into a guilt pit. Could I get back to you in an hour?" And in that hour you may want to call one of your empathy exchange partners, or consult your Giraffe journal. ("Giraffe" is a symbol or nickname for Nonviolent Communication, and the journal is where you record all the wonderful things people have said to you and about you.) Remember that your empathy partners are those people in your support tribe that you call when you are in reaction and need supportive listening to process the reaction. Ideally, it is an equal exchange between yourself and someone else who is learning the art of empathy. Heinze Kohut, the existential psychologist, said that what human beings need most is the mirroring presence of others.

6.   Be quiet, and give yourself a chance to reconnect with the kind of energy and the intention you would like to be coming from, before you respond. (This option can be useful at any of the above points.) You might say to yourself: "I am scared and angry right now. I am going to wait until what I say might help matters."

7.   Be a jackal (the irrational, righteous part of ourselves that takes a position and defends it to the death, that expresses itself as blame, analysis or judgment). Go ahead and be a jerk, but do it with the conscious intent to blow off steam, not cause injury. Even announce your intent. You might say: "This is my jackal voice, trying to free itself, talking here. Quit whining, you pathetic sack of self-pity."

8.   Be a conscious Giraffe Fundalmentalist and give a giraffe lecture like this: "When you are calling someone selfish, you are obviously in judgment, and wanting something for your self! So why is that not selfish?"

Asking an angry "Why?" question is the best way I know of to look like a prosecuting attorney. A Giraffe Fundalmentalist is usually someone who is a recently born-again convert to Nonviolent Communication. They often use the lingo of the process to try to educate or convert others—meanwhile they have, for the moment, lost connection with the spirit of the process, which is compassion. I speak from experience because when I first learned NVC, I used the terminology to defend myself and to attack people. I was much more focused on preaching NVC than I was practicing NVC. As time has passed I have mellowed some and now try to keep my attention more focused on being a compassionate and honest giraffe than trying to get others to be giraffes. But for a long time if someone used language that did not fit the NVC paradigm, for example a label, judgment or exaggeration, I would practically scream at them, "That's violent judgmental communication!" And when they would get angry or hurt in response to my diatribe, I would launch into Giraffe Lecture Mode: "I am not causing your painful feelings. It's what your inner jackal is telling you about what I said that is causing your pain." This was of course a defense from feeling guilty about triggering their anger or hurt.

I recommend the last two options on the above list only as an alternative to becoming self-destructively violent. By self-destructively violent I mean shutting down due to your own thoughts of self-judgment and the resulting feelings of fear, shame, and guilt. These last two can also be a conscious alternative to lashing out in anger with the unconscious intent to create pain.

Decreasing the Danger of Distorting

If you are going to distort or exaggerate something, it is helpful to acknowledge that it is a distortion before you say it. Like, "I know this is an exaggeration, but please hear how it feels in my body. I feel like you are trying to suffocate me." Then take time to unwrap the feelings and needs underneath the distortion. Example: "When you ask me if I am going to come to your party, I feel tense and scared and anxious, because I really need reassurance that if I say no, I will not be punished." In general though, it is better not to use images and exaggerations to build a case for your pain and fear, better to express the needs and feelings behind the distortions in the first place. Say your pain and needs as simply and nakedly as possible.

> If you want to be free of strife,
> Engage yourself in the stream of life,
> By always nakedly revealing
> Your present needs and feelings.

Taking a Step Back

Have you ever gotten a fishing line all tangled up? Then you become so frustrated that you start yanking on the different loops of line, which of course makes the knots even tighter and more difficult to untangle. Would it not be great if you could notice that you were starting to do that in a discussion with your loved one, and were able to stop, take a step back, a time out, before the frustrated yanking occurs? If the time out could be taken before intense anger and frustration occurs, the tangles would not be as difficult to untangle later. And if it could be understood that the request for the time out was in the service of reconnecting with oneself, then the reconnection with the beloved would happen all the sooner. Instead, what I sometimes do is to take space in a huff, implying with my body language and tone that "she is impossible, it is hopeless, and I cannot take any more of this." Often, I am afraid I have only two choices:

a.   To hang in there and yank and struggle and fight until we get through this mess or:

b.   To take space and feel unresolved, disconnected, lonely, worried, unsettled, for hours on end, until we come back and finish the argument.

I am excited about a new option. We can take space in love as an expression of caring for the relationship and in hopes of getting back into connection all the sooner, protecting us from the consequence of making the tangles worse. During that "taking space" time, here are six things I can do:

1. Think about my part of the tangle, to gain clarity about what my reaction was about.

2. Not think at all about the distressing discussion, but enjoy the break from the struggle, trusting that with rest, new energy and clarity will come organically.

3. Translate my jackals first. I do this by feeling into, and naming, the feelings and needs I am having in my body when all that argumentative thinking is going on. Example: my Jackal says, "God, is she controlling!" I feel into my body and translate: "I am feeling irritated, tense, confused and scared because I am wanting to stick up for my needs."

4. Translate her jackals. I do this by thinking about, or writing down, what I think she is feeling and needing behind her words.

5. Turn to music, nature, sports, something totally involving of the mind. (Reading might be difficult.)

6. Write in a journal.

Many of the couples I work with have the following kind of pain going on. The woman is hurt, discouraged, hopeless and lonely while the man is angry, frustrated, exhausted and scared. The woman's unmet need is for empathy, closeness and a higher quality of intimate conversation. The man's need is for respect, rest, validation of his worth as he is, and unhooking himself from his inner sense of guilt and inadequacy about his partner's pain. Again this issue is related to the old freedom v. closeness dance that underlies so many painful relationships. How sad that so many couples spend their whole lives in conflict about this. And it does not even need to be seen as a conflict. (As Einstein said it, "No problem can be solved from the same level of consciousness that created it.") One could look at this freedom v. closeness dynamic not as a conflict but as an important beautiful, playful co-creation. Just as the kite loves its freedom to sail the skies, it still needs the grounding securing quality of the string. The kite stretches the string to new heights, and the string protects the kite from getting lost and

> -§-
> There is no desperation to connect with another person. If I am feeling desperate it is because I have lost connection with me.
> -§-

crashing. It is the dynamic tension between the kite and the string that allows the fulfillment of their different purposes. It is not a conflict to be resolved but a daring, delightful dance, a passionate tango, (not to be mixed up with a tangle) to continually be mastered. Oh, but how to get the word out?

If I were back in my hippie days, I would take off all my clothes, drop some mind-altering, fear-destroying drug, and get two big pieces of cardboard. I would write on one of them in big block letters with oil paint that I stole from the University of Florida Museum of Natural History: "WOMEN! YOU DO NOT HAVE TO GET HIM TO HEAR YOU; YOU JUST NEED TO BE HEARD BY SOMEONE!"

If there is attachment to having a specific person hear your pain, usually several dynamics are set into motion. First, the fear that if your one and only does not hear you, you will stay stuck in the pain; this fear often gets perceived by the other as a compulsive demand or an attack. This is especially true if the fear is not verbalized. Secondly, there is usually some blame mixed in if you think you must be heard by a specific person, who you believe caused the pain. Thirdly, if your significant other buys your belief that he is the only person on the planet that can relieve your pain, and therefore he tries to fill your need to be heard, two things will likely happen:

-§-
Intimacy is found through the balance of freedom and closeness.
-§-

First he will lose the awareness that he has a choice about whether to listen or not and start to perceive your sweet need to be heard as a burden. Second, if he pretends to listen, he will accumulate resentment which he will dump on you later. If you know that your need is for empathy and not empathy *from him,* it makes you less desperate. This will lessen the pressure on him and increase the likelihood he will listen, and listen with more presence.

On the other side of the sandwich board, I would write: "MEN! YOU NEVER HAVE TO LISTEN TO ONE MORE WORD THAN YOU WANT TO HEAR!" For each word you listen to that you did not want to, you will resent her and hold her responsible even though you volunteered for listening duty. And she loses respect every second you are submitting to her instead of being truly present with honesty or empathy. Once I'd donned my message board, I would parade through very densely trafficked areas of the city in hopes of raising the consciousness of the people, so their suffering could end.

I wish that both men and women would refuse to listen to each other unless they were sure it was a compassionate contribution to the other's need to be heard instead of a caving-in concession. May we only "give to" each other and never "give in" to each other lest we breed the slimy serpents of resentment. The pain,

-§-
A "need" is never linked to a specific person or action. It is a universal human condition. That is why it inspires compassion.
-§-

and the emptiness, and the loneliness can become so intense for women that they truly become either desperate or hopeless. They get into aggressive demanding, pleading, or moping around in a slop of self-hate or self-pity, both of which are hard not to interpret as demands. If they could just get some high quality listening and empathy somewhere, it would take some of the charge and intensity off their pain and make it easier to open a dialogue with their mates.

If your partner overwhelms you, or talks your ear off, or "dumps all over you," please notice that you probably chose to sit and take it. Believe me, you did not do her any favor, because you will make her pay for it somehow. Notice too that it was probably not for any great noble reason. It was probably because you were afraid to create conflict, afraid to disturb the image of yourself as a nice person, or you were afraid of losing the other's approval.

Whenever I let my partner do any of the above to me, or otherwise "accidentally oppress" me, I like to apologize to her. I like to tell her about my regret that I let her get her needs met at my expense. I recommit to living "me first and only" so that the love in our relationship will continue to flourish. Then even if I have to use protective force, like running to my room and locking myself in, I will be clear that I am not abandoning the relationship, I am rescuing the relationship. I am rescuing the relationship by not getting caught up in what may very well be the only relationship issue there is: self-abandonment. Not speaking up for yourself is a choice you make to abandon yourself, usually as an attempt to buy love. It never works.

There may be particular pains that your partner cannot empathize with until she resolves certain pains of her own. It is still necessary for you to get that empathy somewhere. It does not mean you need to refrain from asking your partner for empathy about other things. Some men and women are afraid to get heard by someone other than their partner because they interpret this as infidelity or disloyalty. They fear that if they open up their vulnerability and heart to someone else; it will give their partner permission to intimately connect with someone else in a way that could lead to loss. Others think of it as inappropriately airing the family's dirty laundry and are afraid of the family being looked down upon in the community. And of course this does happen in certain communities. Still others are afraid of having their vulnerability trampled upon in the various ways I have already mentioned.

-§-
At those angry moments that I am thinking I want respect, what I really want is empathy to the fear and pain going on in me.
-§-

This kind of "closed system" of communication within the couple-hood creates the same kind of static, stale build-up that occurs when a river is dammed off from its natural refreshing flow. Frustration and irritation gets so built up in a man that a woman's slightest request unleashes the backlog of resentment. His partner may wind up walking on eggshells.

This resentment arises from the man's own self-abandonment. He has listened when he most needed to be heard. He was trying to be strong, rather than resting and recharging when he needed it. He did not know that he had a choice not to listen. Had he known that listening when you need to be heard (or rest) is violence to both partners, he might have avoided the deterioration of the relationship. You violate your responsibility to yourself and begin to hate yourself whenever you do not take care of your own needs. Also you begin to hate and resent the other and hold the illusion that she is oppressing you.

This dynamic sometimes occurs with the genders reversed. But for the sake of simplicity, I will continue to describe it in the way I have more frequently observed in counselling sessions.

Somewhere along the line, the man grows to dread seeing the woman's pain for several reasons:

1.   He interprets it as accusation. His self-talk goes, "I hear your pain. You think I'm not good enough."

2.   He interprets it as proof of his inadequacy. He thinks, "If she is still in pain, I must not be adequately providing for her; therefore I must be inadequate."

3.   He thinks he has no choice but to sit and listen. (We all hate whatever we have no choice about, whether it's lectures from Dad, finishing our broccoli, or paying our taxes.)

4.   It triggers fear that the relationship is ending, which he wants to avoid.

Because men tend to have fear of their own anger about powerlessness, and shame from thinking they are somehow inadequate, sophisticated men learn to go up to their heads to hide behind projective, politically and spiritually correct analytical labels of their partners. Here are a few of my favorites:

1.   "She is just playing victim." Translation: "I am angry that I am choosing to take on responsibility for the pain she is experiencing, and therefore am feeling guilty about it."

2.   "She is so neeeedy." Translation: "I am scared to tell her that I have different needs than she does right now—partly because of the shame I have about having needs at all, but also because I am afraid I will be abandoned if I do not meet her needs."

3.   "She is overly dependent." Translation: "I am confused about how to assert my needs for independence and am tempted to plead with her to please give me permission to be independent. I am unaware that I already have freedom, and I am free to not take care of her."

The woman, on the other hand, often becomes either despondent and despairing about ever getting her needs for support and connection met, or angry thinking he should be willing and able to meet her needs. She begins to resent and fear him for these reasons:

1. She interprets his irritation and frustration about hearing her needs as proof of her "neediness."

2. She interprets his disappointment and depression with his life as "I am not enough to make him happy."

3. She thinks "it's the beginning of the end" and "the other shoe is about to drop."

4. She perceives his pouting and escaping into his cave as rejection or an attempt to gain control in the relationship. Then she begins to take refuge in her judgments of him, often with a little help from her friends:

a. "He is a TAM (Typical Assinine Male), clueless, self-absorbed and out of touch." Translation: "I am frustrated and exasperated about not knowing how to make an emotional connection with him—so he might stay in touch and want to meet my needs."

b. "He is playing the withholding-love control game." Translation: "I am feeling hurt, powerless and confused and want to protect myself from giving in out of my fear of abandonment."

c. "He is being verbally abusive and dominating." Translation: "I am scared and angry. I don't know how to stay present in this situation instead of shrinking from him."

-§-
I am really never afraid of the other's judgment, only of having my own inner self-judgment triggered by their judgment.
-§-

When I enter into an "intensive needs negotiation session" with a loved one (otherwise known as a "fight"), I need to be able to detect the difference between compromise (giving in and giving up) and a true shift, opening the heart to compassion. If I have no confidence that I can make this distinction, I will be too scared to really listen, empathize and take in what the other person is expressing. I am afraid that I may feel sorry for them—and end up giving in when I don't want to. Then I will have to deal with self-hate. (My inner Jackal saying, "Wimp, people pleaser, why do you let people push you around!") Or with resentment. (Inner Jackal: "Why

do they always have to have their way? They are selfish! It is not fair!")
It is this fear of self-abandonment that contributes to the fear of hearing what the other is really saying. Another fear that gets in my ear is about taking in something that will trigger self-judgment, shame or guilt.

When I have no feeling sense that the other is empathizing with my expression of needs, it is very easy to interpret their expressions of having a different need as an attack. When I am not feeling that energy of connection, understanding and acceptance, *or when I have low energy,* it is easy to misinterpret what the other is saying as a criticism of me. Example:

My beloved says: "I have felt disconnected and alone for days now."

I hear: "You unconscious creep. What kind of beloved are you? How could you let me suffer so? Your companionship is inadequate."

I am then very tempted to lash out with something like, "Well, if you would just get a life, then you would not feel so lonely!" Of course, the reason I feel so defensive is because I feel guilty, and I've chosen to protect myself from that feeling by getting angry. Obviously I am not teflon-coated on that issue: I still have an inner Jackal that believes I am guilty — or else the accusation wouldn't stick to me and need defending. I am reminded of two *Ruminations,* which are little one-liners that a whimsical part of me thinks I channel from the ancient mystic poet Rumi. (*Rumi-Nations* — coming soon to a bookstore near you.) Rumination #1: "If a judgment sticks, it is still yours." Rumination #2, for my poor partner who has to deal with how I hear her express her needs to me: "You express your sweet needs to me, and I then add them to my list of inadequacies."

-§-
You tell me your sweet needs, and I add them to my list of inadequacies
-§-

This behavior of lashing out in verbal or physical violence stems from the fear of, or the perception of, being attacked. My beloved could greatly reduce the likelihood that I will perceive attack if she makes connection with me, or empathizes with my fear, before she shares her needs and her pain. If she has not waited so long that she is in a lot of pain she might be able to approach me gently. She might start with something like this: "My sense is that you have been preoccupied with work, or maybe you've been feeling a little down these last several days. Is that true?" I say "Yup." She says, "Well I have been missing you and would like to reconnect somehow. Would you be willing to talk about how we might do that?" Notice her emphasis on the present moment and meeting present needs. Nonviolent Communication is always based in this very moment. Even if I want to spend some time with you in the future, I want the agreement to do so to happen now.

When I imply or tell someone that what they did was wrong (Example: "Everybody is more important to you than me!"), I am often motivated by two fearful beliefs. First, that I am going to be judged (as selfish or needy) for asserting my need at all. Second, because I think that I don't deserve to have my needs met in the first place, it becomes important to "make a case" against the other. I believe I need to prove that the other's behavior "caused" my suffering and so restitution is now owed.

I am also hoping to protect myself from feeling guilty by holding the other totally responsible for my pain and unmet needs. This prevents me from becoming conscious of my part in the interaction and allows me to stay stuck in a feeling reality of powerlessness. Another part of me is hoping that if I make a compelling case that you were motivated by evil forces, you will have no credibility when you defend yourself by calling me "overly sensitive," "partially responsible" and so on.

Fears that my needs will not be responded to with compassion become self-fulfilling prophecies.

Searching for Synergistic Solutions

In order to get good at finding synergistic solutions, it is important to develop a consciousness and a language for expressing needs, instead of only being able to identify and express requests. If I can only express the behavior change I want to see in the future, it looks to you like I am locked into my one and only way to get the need met. This can easily trigger your fear of being taken advantage of, which leads to power struggles.

This is sometimes called "singlemindedness of purpose." It usually generates resistance. A better intention is to establish a feeling sense of connection and a deep understanding of everyone's needs. From this connection, trust, goodwill and grace can inspire the cooperation and creativity needed to get everyone's needs met peacefully. I have seen it happen every single time that people make a sincere effort. Dr. Rosenberg calls this result *inevitable,* and my experience confirms this.

-§-
The issue will take care of itself once the intimacy is established.
-§-

When both parties are locked into "request consciousness" it looks like there is no way to get both requests met. This is when fear arises and each party starts to pull for their request in whatever ways they were taught in their family. The two most popular strategies are "power over" (saying or doing things that evoke shame or fear to coerce the other to give in) and "power under" (saying or doing something to trigger guilt to coerce the other to give in).

Example of "request consciousness":

John: "Jane, I need you to stay home tonight."

Jane: "And I need you to quit being so controlling."

Translation into "needs consciousness":

John: "I am feeling restless and need to have some company and play. Would you brainstorm with me about what I or we might do tonight?"

Jane: "I am worried about giving in. I am also confused about what I want to do tonight. I need to get clearer within myself—so I would like to think about it for maybe ten minutes and get back to you. Would that work for you?"

"Needs consciousness" opens the door to thousands of solutions and makes it easier for the other to trust that you do not have your mind all made up. It also makes it easier to trust that there is room in the solution for everyone involved to get their needs met. This process is like a game of "connect the dots," with the needs being the dots. And by needs I mean universal general needs, without mention of any specific people or actions (because specific actions are requests not needs). The more clear the needs (dots) we put on the page, the easier it is to see the big picture that is the solution to the problem. It is important that we get needs expressed as clearly as possible before we try to move to solution (*connecting* the dots) or else we will not produce a whole picture. It is also sometimes helpful to remember what it says at the bottom of the page in the newspaper crossword puzzle section: "The answer to today's puzzle will appear in tomorrow's edition."

Just expressing feelings and requests is not nearly as effective as expressing feelings, needs and requests. Example of feelings and requests:

John: "I am feeling frustrated. Will you stay home tonight?"

Example of feelings, needs and requests:

John: "I am feeling frustrated, and really wanting some company. Would you be willing to stay home tonight?"

Almost all the power to inspire compassion comes from expressing the need, and only a little from expressing the feeling. Also when I am listening to someone, it is much more powerful to demonstrate that I understand the other's need than it is to just show that I have heard his feeling and request. Example:

John: "I want you to stay home tonight."

Jane: "Are you feeling frustrated and want company?"

This is much more likely to create a sense of connection and understanding than:

John: "I want you to stay home tonight."

Jane: "Are you feeling frustrated and want me to stay home?"

If I hear just the person's feelings, he will likely keep repeating himself until he gets the sense that his needs are being heard.

Freedom v. Closeness

Now I will write about a subject that is so volatile and controversial that you might want to burn this book after reading it. It is an aspect of that deepest of male/female conflicts, the freedom need v. the closeness need.

One battleground this plays out on is the traditional monogamous marriage versus the open, non-monogamous marriage. Neither monogamy nor non-monogamy are needs. They are both strategies, i.e. requests for specific actions. I recommend that couples learn how to talk deeply and thoroughly about the needs behind these requests. Here are some of the needs that lie behind the strategy of monogamy:

Closeness
Interdependence
Emotional security
Simplicity
Focus on depth of relationship
Consistency
Peace of mind that comes from following one's convictions
Financial security
Social security

Here are some of the needs that lie behind the strategy of non-monogamy:

Freedom
Autonomy
Exploration of different parts of oneself
Aliveness
Community
Integrity with self
Openness
Pleasure
Interdependence
Spiritual growth

Serious problems might be avoided if each person thought about these needs and how they relate to their personal view of marriage. From that clarity, a discussion could either stop the marriage or else make it stronger, depending on the understandings involved. This is not the only arena in which Freedom v. Closeness plays out in relationships, but it is a big one. Other issues might involve whether or not to call about being "late," how often to visit families, passionate hobbies not shared, etc.

If couples can take responsibility for their needs and learn to negotiate them using "need language," what was a conflict becomes a lovemaking session. One of the reasons conflict is scary is because we live in an androcratic Domination Culture (male dominated), and the way most conflict is dealt with is through control, violent force and punishment to maintain the order and power of those presently in charge. However within a couplehood, we can create a loving mini-culture that does not require any one person to be in charge, and therefore no one has to give in or be oppressed. I say this because finding ways to meet each other's needs without compromising ourselves is one of my favorite definitions of love.

If a couple is locked into conflict about any specific request, I recommend they go back to hearing each other on the need level. Scene 1: Husband and wife are entering into a fight:

Husband: "Look, why are you being so paranoid? I am sure we can afford to buy the boat now."

Wife: "No we can't. Besides you are never home as it is. If you get a boat I will never see you."

Husband: "Well, if you would get a life, you would not resent me for wanting to have a little boating fun. And we can too afford it."

Wife: "No, we can't."

This is where it is helpful to slow down, back up, and start listening for the needs behind the request. In Scene 2 the wife wakes up and decides to use her Nonviolent Communication skills to get connected on the need level. Scene 2: Wife leads dialogue into an "intensive needs negotiation session."

Wife: "I am scared about where this is heading. Let me see if I can really hear your needs for getting the boat and getting it now. Are you wanting a boat because you are wanting to reward yourself for all the hard work you have been doing? And do you want to get it now because you are afraid you will resent missing the sailing season if you wait any longer?"

Husband: "No, the sailing season is already over. I am wanting a boat because I am hitting 50, and I want some adventure in my life before I die. I want it now because I am afraid it will get put on the back burner again, and I don't know how long my health is going to be good."

Wife: "So you are worried about having some excitement while you can still enjoy it?"

Husband: "Yes, thank you for hearing that."

Husband (moved by her generosity of spirit at trying to empathize with his needs): "So let me see now if I can hear you. Are you worried that we will run out of money before our daughter gets through college? Like a need to know your child will be OK?"

Wife: "To be honest with you that is only a small part of it. The bigger part is probably my fear of being alone all the time."

Husband: "So are you afraid and need to trust that your needs for companionship will get met?"

Wife: "Yeah. Something like that."

Husband: "Well, I have needs for companionship too. What say I make you first mate and we sail off together into the sunset?"

Wife: "That sounds great, honey, except that you know I don't know how to sail. And you get so crabby whenever you try to teach me something. Remember the computer?"

Husband: "But that was before we learned NVC. Oops! Sorry about that. I just put my "but" in your face. Let me try again. Are you scared that we will get into the kinds of fights we did around the computer, and are you needing reassurance that you will be taught how to sail with gentleness and patience?"

Wife: "Yes, but I don't know how to get the reassurance."

Husband: "Well, I would like you to notice how we just now navigated through these stormy waters. You were great applying NVC to bring us back into connection with each others needs. I am sure that if you can keep having patience with my process of learning NVC, I can have patience as I teach you how to set a course for some smooth sailing."

Each of us is ultimately responsible for our own needs. If we become exhausted trying unsuccessfully to negotiate a need with a particular person, we still will need to take care of it somehow. The freedom need is a special need, in that it cannot be obtained from your partner or anyone else. It is a gift only you can give you.

A part of meeting a need for freedom is learning how to steer clear of the pothole of guilt. One way out of guilt is to really hear the other's pain. When we are feeling guilty we are still resisting empathizing with the other's pain. We are not yet one with their pain. When I am one with the other's pain, there are no feelings of guilt or defensiveness.

One of the reasons people do not get along is because they interpret each other's quest for freedom as an attempt to limit their own. When there is trust in the basic compassion of human beings, the escalating Ping-Pong of distrust and protection through attack does not occur. When there is a value of really trying to minimize the impact I make on you in my quest for freedom, and a willingness to seek solutions that will create the least impact for both of us, even while supporting the most freedom for both of us, we might be able to get along. It is only the fear that I might have to give up my freedom, (as I remember pain from prisons past) that prevents me from having empathy for your pain from my impact on you.

If the idea of my freedom scares you, it is probably because of your prediction that I will use my freedom to neglect you and your pain from past trauma. The more true freedom we have, the less likely we are to try to get our needs met at anyone's expense. This is true partly because the more freedom we have, the more options we have for getting our needs met in other places. Violence and taking advantage of others often comes out of desperation, powerlessness, and a fear that there are no other options. One big reason people separate or leave a relationship is because they fear there is no way to get their needs met or have the freedom they want while continuing to stay in the relationship. After years of believing they need to compromise their needs for freedom in order to have security, the pain and resentment leads them to *break* free.

However, there is no such thing as a need to compromise. Compromise is a strategy with the intention to keep harmony. But the general outcome of compromise is to divide up the resentment fifty-fifty. When we act with the intention of not giving in, we catalyze satisfying and synergistic solutions. Plus we create a context for "giving to" the other person.

Avoid shorthand words like "messy" or "lazy" or "cranky" about each other's behavior, until you have developed the level of trust to know that these words are banter, not judgment. It adds joyful color to kid my partner, "My, my, aren't you a little cranky this morning!" Because there is a history of building trust, my beloved can hear me saying, "When you growl at me on the way to the bathroom like that, I am concerned that you may be feeling out of sorts this morning. Would you like to talk about it?"

What Love is *Not*

Some feelings and needs I choose to suppress. Like when the policeman pulls me over and I choose to put my anger into the refrigerator rather than express it. Once he is gone I can take it out of the refrigerator and revel in my rage. I want to be careful not to repress, by putting it into the freezer, trying to forget about it and hope it goes away. That is what happened to us as children and now all that rotten stuff is unthawing. Suppression can be a very life serving-action, as it is a channeling of emotional energy to meet certain needs. Suppression=Refrigerator.

Repression moves emotional energy into the unconscious where it will fester until it bursts out in destructive unconscious expression.

Repression=Freezer. Repression is where we ignore certain feelings (usually "negative" ones like anger, sadness, fear, shame, and so on). Or we ignore needs (usually ones that have been culturally shamed like sex, rest, play, and even ones that are less easily recognized: empathy (big kids don't cry), self-expression (stop showing off!) and community (oh, look, the little boy is lonely).

Rebellion=The fear of submission. If I think I have to choose between submission and rebellion, I will choose rebellion.

In my private practice as a marriage therapist I am forever getting one member of a couple or maybe both coming to me separately saying that they are seriously considering leaving the relationship. When I ask them why, they say it is because this need or that is not getting met. When I check to see if they are clearly asking for their needs, I find out that they are not. I usually suggest that they go ahead and ask for whatever it is since there is so little to lose.

Invariably the litany of excuses start to flow: "It is no use. I am sure she would not go for it. I do not want to upset her." Or "What if he leaves me? If he loved me he would know what I want and give it to me without my having to ask." Or "I cannot deal with the rejection if she says no"… and so on. Of course it is this fear-based, static thinking that prevented a flow of negotiation which might have made the relationship work.

Much better to go ahead and ask for everything you want and let the chips fall where they may. Practice being your full, authentic self in the face of your fear of abandonment. If you cannot do it in a relationship that you are not sure you want to keep, you surely will not be able to do it in one that you do want to keep.

I sometimes ask a couple to express their needs to each other this way: I might say, "Okay, Sue, ask Bob this question: 'How can I make your life richer?'" She asks him.

Bob answers: "Give me a divorce."

Me: "What are your needs behind your request for a divorce?"

Bob: "I don't know, I am not happy. She won't accept me as I am. She's always criticizing me about something, complaining or being paranoid. The sex has become boring, and we just have different needs."

The more I investigate, often the clearer it is that neither person is clearly expressing his or her needs. Usually they are expressing their pain through culturally-assigned, gender-role language and images: the wife as victim and slave, the husband as perpetrator and master.

Sometimes I will playfully tell them, "Look, you see your relationship as shot anyway, so you might as well use it as target practice. By that I mean you may as well practice clearly asking for everything you want since there is nothing to lose anyway." I offer a guarantee that if they do this, there will be either a breakthrough or a breakdown. If you create a breakthrough, great, you are on the road again. If you create a breakdown, great, then you can give each other a compassionate divorce, wish each other well, and maybe even give each other the gift of moving to opposite sides of the planet. I consider that either will likely be a relief, far preferable to the slow, painful death they are currently experiencing.

> -§-
> The better we can relate together, the better we can create together.
> -§-

Sometimes I get extremely frustrated and angry thinking "I need respect. I am not being respected!" However, when I really take the time to look at what is going on in me, I see that often I am scared and needing a sense of connection that could occur if I got reassurance that my needs are understood in the situation. And concretely asking for this reassurance sounds far less threatening than "demanding respect" in a vague way.

From a "me first and only" perspective it is easier to be an equal and create equality in the relationship. And at the same time, it is becoming clearer that the more fiercely protective I am of my partner's needs, the more I benefit, and the more equality I create.

What does "love our enemies" mean? Is it an oxymoron? By definition you are not loving someone if you are seeing them as an enemy. Anyone you are seeing or thinking about as an enemy you are afraid of, and fear is the opposite of love. For me love is an action, not a psychological state. It is not an emotion that I can whip up on demand. So for me to love someone I was previously thinking of as an enemy, I need to understand and have empathy for whatever is going on in her behind her actions that I have found disturbing. In relationships, the whole idea of vanquishing the enemy is psychologically bankrupt. I must vanquish the "enemy" images in my head before my heart can open to the truth of the human being in front of me. To do this I must get conscious of the needs in my own body underneath the "enemy" images (like "terrorist," "evil" person, "attacker," "insensitive" person, "violent" person, "unconscious" person) in my head.

Love of enemies is both a spiritual path and a process of psychological healing and maturing. It requires that we stop projecting our hate of our own disowned parts onto others and humbly accept and integrate those shadow parts. Instead of judging someone as selfish we accept the part of ourselves that gets scared at times and would horde. We then extend that understanding to the other. This does not require us to condone it. Indeed, I would use nonviolent actions to protect myself from loss and to free the other person from the painful dynamics of acting oppressively.

In Walter Wink's book *Jesus and Nonviolence,* he says this:

> Love of enemies has, for our time, become the litmus test of authentic Christian faith. Commitment to justice, liberation, or the overthrow of oppression is not enough, for all too often the means used have brought in their wake new injustices and oppressions. Love of enemies is the recognition that the enemy, too, is a child of God.

What a timely reminder in this post 9/11 world. I believe that all the violent solutions in the world will never produce radical enough changes to bring us the sense of safety we want. To twist a phrase from Wink's book "Either we find the God who causes the sun to rise on the terrorists (them: the evil enemies) and on the liberators (us: the good guys), or we may have no more sunrises."

When we judge another, we not only stop thinking about possible solutions—thus increasing the likelihood we will resort to some form of violence, we also place the other in a position of inferiority in our minds. This attitude makes it easier to mistreat them with impunity.

This justification-thinking happens at all levels of society. I recently heard President George W. Bush say that our enemies do not understand reason, only military force. This of course is the old tactic of suggesting that a whole group of people is somehow missing an essential quality of humanness. Dehumanizing them is a prerequisite step to discrimination or extermination. The Nazis spoke of the Jews as inferior, white supremacists claim blacks to be sub-human animals, and American pioneers saw the Indians as savages, which made it easier to kill them and take their land.

So just as we cannot "demand" respect from another, (a disrespectful act in itself) and obtain real respect, we cannot use violence to inspire the respect upon which real democracy is built. However, I can command respect first by refusing to see the other as anything less than a divine being with human feelings and needs. Secondly, I can hold onto my dignity by remembering that I too am an innocent being only trying to get my human needs met. This protects me from psychological violence and provides me with "projection protection."

If I defend myself from the other's projection, they feel justified in their projection. If I empathize with their projection, they are left owning it. It is exhausting to play passive doormat in the name of trying to be holy; it spiritually wears us out. However, it is invigorating to take up hearts (rather than arms) and create a divine dialogue designed to include the other person in the solution.

Finally, when we stay current, we keep a loving current flowing. Staying current means expressing resentments, hurts, angers, celebrations, joys, losses, appreciations and irritations to your partner as soon as there is a space for them.

You've heard of the Golden Rule, "Do unto others as you would have them do unto you." It assumes that others want the same thing you do in every situation. A more evolved love is less self centered, demonstrating empathy to the unique needs of others. How about the Platinum Rule: "Do unto others as they would have themselves done unto."

What Love Is Not
by Kelly Bryson

Love is not saying "I love you" when your lover is thirsty;
It is giving them a drink.
Love is not hugging your sunburned lover;
It is rubbing them with lotion made of zinc.
Love is not reading her a love poem
When she is trying to go to sleep.
It is giving her your precious absence,
That shows your love runs deep.
So if you love them, you will leave them when they need to rest.
Otherwise you will become a kind of lover's pest.
If you want to make a mess,
Always say yes.
If you want love to go,
Never say no.

Releasing the Pressure

If I perceive pressure from people, I am not hearing them. My own autonomy has been hooked and I am now in fear. I need empathy to my own fear before I can really hear their urgency. Also, if I can empathize with the other's urgency or fear of not getting his needs met, this will greatly decrease the likelihood he will hear my "no" as a rejection. For example: Someone runs up to you at a dance and grabs your hand and starts to pull you onto the dance floor. You are uncomfortable dancing with this person at the moment. You might respond: "So you are really wanting to dance? And I am just wanting to watch for the moment."

If the other senses a heart-connection between us, she won't perceive our "no" as a lack of caring. This makes it easier for her to hear that the "no" is just us taking care of ourselves, not a rejection of her. Our empathy to her urgency helps her feel accurately received. Giving someone empathy before we tell them "No" takes the sting out of what might be perceived as a rejection.

A frequent misperception of intention happens when I think someone is "trying to pressure me," and I interpret his motive as trying to get his needs met at my expense. When I think this way, there is often a look of suspicion in my eye that is likely to trigger all the more hurt and panic for the other. How reassuring to him if I can first empathize with my own fear, taking a moment to be present to my own reaction. Then I can give empathy from my heart.

Needs are never in conflict. Only solutions or requests can be in conflict. For example being hungry and tired are two needs. They are not really in conflict until I try to make a request of myself like to go to a restaurant or take a nap. These requests are in conflict. If I can let go of making a decision for a moment, and just be with my needs, the decision will make me. As I feel into my need for rest and nutrition, I will either fall asleep, or decide to recline with a snack, or eat a TV dinner before resting, or ask my partner to make me some food as I rest.

Love is never having to say or do anything. If I think I have to or must do something for someone, I am submitting. What I am doing is not coming freely from me and therefore is not love.

Compassionate Comebacks

John : "Hi, Mary. Long time no see. How about a hug?"

Mary: "Get away from me, you codependent, parasitic pest. You are not roping me into another sick, twisted, controlling relationship!"

John: "Thank you. I can see now that it would be very scary for you to hug me right now."

Mary: "You got that right, buster."

John: "And you would like to protect yourself from the kind of pain and control you have experienced in past relationships?"

Mary: "That's for sure."

John: "I assume you would like to get to know me better before having a hug?"

Mary: "Yes."

John: "Longer than the twelve years we have known each other?"

If men could express their fear when they felt it, instead of worrying about being wimps, and women could be true to themselves instead of worrying about being thought of as bitchy, the world would sweeten up and the streets would be safe.

It is more difficult to stay in sweet, deep dialogue with people you really care about than with mere acquaintances for these reasons:

1. It is more difficult to see them in pain, or allow them to have their pain, because you don't want them to suffer.

2. The potential loss, if they get upset and leave, is greater.

3. Your heart is on the line.

If we empathize with the other person's reaction when he misinterprets our intention as an attack, we can restore his sense of safety. It is helpful to practice empathizing with people's misinterpretations of our intentions. Here are some typical ones, with compassionate comebacks:

Statement: "You're just in this venture for the money."

Compassionate Comeback: "Are you worried and would like an explanation of my motives?"

Statement: "You are trying to take advantage of me."

Compassionate Comeback: "Are you scared and wanting some reassurance that you are cared about?"

Statement: "You meant to hurt my feelings!"

Compassionate Comeback: "Are you angry and wanting honesty about my motives for saying what I did?"

Statement: "You do not care about me."

Compassionate Comeback: "Are you feeling hurt and needing some indication that you do matter?"

Statement: "You are trying to manipulate me."

Compassionate Comeback: "Are you feeling distrustful and needing some time to think about the offer I made on your car?"

The Integrity of Interrupting

A conversation is not a marriage. Does proper etiquette demand that whoever begins the conversation, or takes the floor first, is allowed to talk the others into the ground? Many people use words as walls of protection and can get terribly wounded if you "interrupt" them. By "interrupt" I mean say anything while they are still speaking. The reason they get so wounded is because they have an ethnocentric belief (unlike cultures that have no concept of "interrupt") that it is impolite to interrupt others, that one should wait until the other is finished before speaking. So if anyone tries to get a word in edgewise while they are speaking, the Babbleonian (the person using more words than you know how to enjoy) is going to judge them as impolite. These Babbleonians are usually quite oblivious to how overbearing and oppressive their energy is to others. They are often quite empty, scared and lonely because of the isolation their wall of words creates for them. This leaves them with very little awareness of or connection with others and makes them use all the more words, trying to feel heard or seen.

Other times people are unaware of the need that is causing them to speak. They might launch into a story without giving you any indication of why they are telling you the story. If you sit there and listen politely, without interrupting, awaiting your escape, you will resent them and somehow make them pay for "accidentally oppressing" you. The longer you wait to speak up for yourself, the more pain, irritation and fear will be in your voice. It will also become more and more difficult to respond with dignity, grace and power. Example:

Joe: "My dog Charlie was the best old hound anybody ever had. We used to take the best walks out across the canyon. I remember the time..."

Bill: "Excuse me, Joe, I am wondering if you are really missing your old dog Charlie?"

Joe: "Am I ever."

As soon as you are connected with the feeling and need behind the story you will not be bored anymore. You will be connected with the other person's life energy, which will bring you both back to life, and the present.

So one purpose of interrupting is to be sure you, too, are getting your needs for conversation met. It is to create a win/win conversation and not a they win/you lose conversation. Often when I interrupt for the purpose of understanding the speaker, they feel much more heard.

Some people confuse being a good waiter with being a good listener. Just sitting there feeling confused, trying to understand the speaker, is a form of not listening. Waiting patiently and politely for the speaker to finish does not help the speaker feel heard. Waiting for the speaker to inhale, so you can jump in, decreases the likelihood of a quality connection. Besides, some people are capable of speaking on both the inhale and the exhale.

A funny way to frame this situation is to say, "If I was not listening, then speaking up is not technically an interruption of dialogue." I am interrupting a monologue to restore the communication into a dialogue. By interrupting, I am actually helping the speaker get their need for communication met. I am restoring the purpose of communication: to fill the need for connection and accurate understanding.

If you do catch yourself trying to listen when you are on overload, you may want to warn the speaker that each additional word will cost her time and a half for overtime rates. For each word you listen to beyond your limit, you build resentment toward, and lose respect for, the speaker. It's better to stop pretending to listen, and interrupt that person, while you still like him.

Fairly often, no matter how many times I guess, and how hard I try to feel a part of the conversation, I am not able to. So after I have tried a few unsuccessful attempts to guess what the Babbleonian is feeling and needing or requesting of me, I change gears and use honesty instead of empathy. Example:

Joe: "…And then in '62 old Charlie came down with a bad case of mange and we took him to the vet. But the vet was not in his office that day so we took old Charlie…"

Bill: "Excuse me Joe, I am confused, could you tell me what you are wanting from me about old Charlie?"

Joe: "Nothing, I am just telling a story. Why do you have to get so psychological on me?"

Bill: "Okay, Joe, if you are not wanting anything from me about the story, do you mind if I read the newspaper as you tell it?"

If I have let the Babbleonian go on too long, I want to remember to:

1.   Grieve the loss of time and the abandonment of self.

2.   Understand what made me choose to abandon myself, and do this without any self-judgment.

3.   Rededicate myself to being real and honest in each moment.

4.   I might read this poem I wrote, entitled "If You Have a Need, Speak Up With Speed" to remind me to not abandon myself again.

> If you have a need, speak up with speed.
> 'Cause if you don't, you probably won't.
> As soon as you think if you should or you shouldn't,
> You turn your could into a couldn't;
> And as your need you start to swallow,
> Notice your body starts to feel hollow.
> And the more you try to analyze
> The more of your self you paralyze.
> As all the attention drains up to your head,
> The rest of your body is left feeling dead.

Tuning Into Tones

When we are upset with someone's tone we are really in need of connection to that person's feelings. It is just a strategy, and not a need, to ask them to change or lower their tone. Being requested to lower one's voice, or tone it down can easily be heard as "You should stuff your feelings, or your feelings are too much." This is particularly true if the need behind the request is not made clear. If you do decide to ask someone to lower her voice, be sure to also express your need to "feel centered," or "hear her more easily," or "be more present," or something similar. Instead of asking your partner to soften his tone, try asking for him to express what he is saying in terms of his feelings and needs. I have found this often meets the need for safety and connection that the request to lower the tone is trying to meet.

Don and Jim had made a commitment with each other not to raise their voices to each other in public, and they were constantly catching each other breaking the agreement. They were also using the word "rage" as an accusation. "You had rage in your voice now, did you not? Admit it!" I told them I was worried that their commitment was not helping them get to the roots of the problem. I explained that a relationship can be like two gardens that we combine to make one. We cannot really commit to never having weeds sprout in the garden but we can commit to how we are going to deal with them. Anger, rage, contempt, disgust, are all like the tops of dandelion weeds. The roots are hurt, shame, guilt, and fear. In my relationships we are committed to pulling the weeds out by the roots, getting to whatever the pain is really all about underneath the weeds of sarcasm, blame, attempts to punish, demands, or judgment.

-§-
Rumi-nation: "Whenever I say to you 'that's your stuff,' that's my stuff."
-§-

Don: "I had the hardest time getting him to admit that what he said to me was inappropriate."

Me: "I wonder if you were just really feeling hurt in relation to what he said and wanted understanding for that hurt."

Don: "Yeah."

Me: "I am concerned about even thinking that what he said was inappropriate, because it makes it so much harder to get the empathy you are wanting. I do not have any moral judgment on the use of the word 'inappropriate,' nor do I think it is unspiritual, or non-religious. It is just more holistically selfish, more likely to get you what you are wanting, to speak to his compassion. You are less likely to trigger his defensiveness if you were to say that you are hurting now and need understanding for that pain, instead of trying to get him to admit he is being inappropriate."

Don: "OK, I will try it."

I talked with Don a little later and he shared with me the following "giraffe tale"—a story about someone using Nonviolent Communication to a wonderful conclusion. Don and Jim were in a restaurant when the following conversation occurred. They were talking and got caught up in their usual heated political discussion.

Jim (with angry raised voice and tone): "I can not believe what a thick-headed Democrat you are. You never budge on anything!"

Don first became furious, thinking Jim should not talk to him in that inappropriate manner. He gave himself empathy and then said: "Jim, I am feeling irritated and embarrassed right now, because I am wanting to be treated with more respect, especially in public. Would you lower your voice?"

Jim: "No, I won't lower my voice. This is still America and I still have a right to express myself!"

Don, having expressed his feelings, needs, and requests, felt more centered. He was then able to empathize with Jim: "So you're irritated because you want to maintain your right to free speech?"

Jim: "Darn right!"

Don: "I support you in your free speech. Would you please help me with my embarrassment by lowering your voice, or if you need to express yourself this loudly, let's go somewhere else."

Jim: "You're just trying to avoid the fact that you are wrong about Republicans."

Don: "So you distrust my motive in asking us to take the conversation outside?"

Jim now began to naturally lower his voice as he sensed the respect Don was giving him. Jim: "Yeah a little bit. Do you promise to take it up exactly where we left off if we drop it for now?"

Don: "Here, I will write a note on this napkin so we will remember where we left off."

Jim: "Okay, that works for me. And, by the way, thanks for not pointing out what a jerk I was being just now."

Keys for Fun Fighting

Sometimes couples get caught up in a game of trying to get each other to own their stuff. When either one does that, they are subtly trapped in their own judgments. A way out of this is to quit saying, "I want you to own your stuff" and instead start taking responsibility for one's own part. Another rumination I wrote to help me do this is "Anytime I tell you 'that's your stuff,' that's my stuff." If I am labeling someone's expression as 'stuff,' I have slipped back into my old label-game habit, which I do not value. Also I am not taking responsibility to express my own needs, feelings and requests.

When I sense my partner will give me anything I ask for if I threaten to withhold my love, it is very tempting to use this power. Also when I put all my emotional eggs in one basket, one person, it is very difficult for me to stay true to myself when they withhold love from me. If I have many resources, my partner threatening to withhold love or sex has no power over me. And when my partner has other resources for love, I know my withholding will not get her to give in. And besides I want to break out of my "withholding patterns" and develop my negotiating (some would call it fighting) skills. Here are some keys to success for fun fighting:

1.   Good Referees. These are conscious, intimate friends who care about and know both of you well. They need to have a good sense of knowing when to offer empathy, when to offer honesty, and when to butt out.

2.   Friends. People who supply a rich supply of intimacy, to protect against dependency, and the control battles that go with it.

3.   Body Awareness. Developing a keen inner sense of what your body feels like when you are shifting to compassion, versus compromising and giving in.

4.   Focus on Feelings. Having an understanding with your loved ones that when things get intense, it is valuable to quit talking about the content of the argument, and talk just about emotions and needs.

5.   Never Argue Reality. Let each person have his own reality. Instead of saying, "I did not say that!" you might say, "I do not remember saying that."

6.   Don't Fight Beyond the Fun. When a strong wind is tearing the fabric of the sail in your sailboat, it's better to bring the sails down for a while. When the fight has lost all of its fun and is starting to tear at the fabric of the relationship, take a separate time out to journal, take a long walk or process with a friend.

7.   Get Clear First. When in pain, wait till you are clear about what you want back from your partner before you share your pain.

-§-
How does one perfect their victimhood? Ask not what you can do for yourself, ask what is wrong with your partner.
-§-

Then make a do-able request for the empathy, honest, agreements, acknowledgment, appreciation, or information you need. If you just share your pain without making it clear what you want said or done in response, you will likely be seen as an emotional terrorist. An example: "I feel sad that you didn't call me," followed by a long pause with sad eyes. It's more effective to say: "I'm feeling sad; I would have liked some company last night. I need empathy." Then either, "How do you feel about what I am saying?" (honesty), or, "What was going on for you?" (information), or, "Will you call me tomorrow?" (agreements), or "What are you hearing me say?" (empathy).

8.   Once things get heated, refuse to continue to talk about the right/wrong content of the argument and insist on talking about the process. Share the feelings you are having right now about what is happening between the two of you. Make your best guess about what the other is presently feeling and needing about what is happening between you both. Go for the Vulnerability. Drop down out of your head and into your body.

Danger Signals

You know it's time for a pause when you find yourself in any of the following situations:

1.   When your mind tells you: "Ask not what you can do for yourself, ask what is wrong with your partner."

2.   When your mind tells you: "If I can just get her to change her behavior everything will be fine." No amount of control will substitute for trust.

3.   You suddenly feel totally compelled for some unconscious reason to triple you spouse's life insurance.

4.   You are in the check out line at the grocery store and notice you are purchasing the super industrial size bag of Cheetos, a box of 82 jars of chocolate syrup that you told the stock boy not to bother cutting open, and enough ice cream to open a parlor.

5.   You keep putting your "but" in the face of your partner's pain. The partner keeps trying to get you to hear, and you keep saying "Yes, but..."

6.   You or your partner are smiling as anger, sadness or pain is being expressed (or going verbally unexpressed).

7.   You keep moving to solutions (like, "Forget it then, let's end the relationship") before you are conscious of all the needs that seem to be in conflict.

8.   When the quality of connection between the human beings involved seems less important than getting someone to pick up his clothes.

Chapter

THE ECSTASY OF EMPATHY

When I empathize with someone, I become a strong and gentle wind, filling the sails of the other's inner exploration. As the wind, I have no control over the steering of the boat. That is left up to the captain of the ship, the person I am being present to. I do not try to direct, only to connect with where the other is in this very present moment. I bring in no ideas or thoughts about the past or the future. I bring in no thoughts of my own. I have no preference for where we go on this journey—only that it come from the captain's heart and choice. The purpose of my presence is connection, never correction. I am a steady, present trade wind, not an impatient and gusty gale.

Dear Wind
by Donovan

Dear wind that shakes the barley free.
Blow home my true love's ship to me.
Fill her sails.
I wait a weary wait upon the shore.
Protect her oaken beams from harm.
Protect her mast in times of storm.

> Fill her sails.
> I wait a weary wait upon the shore.

Empathy brings in nothing from the past. When I am empathizing I am not remembering when I was having a similar experience. In one sense I am not even there. The only thing present is the other person's experience, feelings and story. I am not relating to the experience, feelings and story themselves; I am being with the felt sense of them. Relating to another's experience is about you. Empathizing is about them.

Some people get so caught up in the fear of wondering whether they are empathizing correctly that very little energy for attention is left to be present with the other.

It is not really *doing* empathy or *giving* empathy — it is *being* empathy. It is the spirit that actress Susan Sarandon exemplifies in the movie "Dead Man Walking." In this film, based on a true story, a man to whom she has served as spiritual advisor is being executed for murder. Susan's character, a nun, wants to be in the viewing room so that her face will be the last thing he sees as he faces death. She wants to be the face of love for her friend.

Empathy is an energy, not a modality or a technique. Empathy is closely related to presence. The following is from the anthology *Healers on Healing,* in an article called "Presence" by Don H. Johnson:

> The dazzling successes of the great teachers and therapists and the unfamiliar quality of their presence have led to a mistaken belief that their success lies in their techniques. Moshe Feldenkrais watched people moving their limbs, paying close attention to what they actually did in a non-judgmental way: this is the essence of therapy…. Although Zen teacher Suzuki Roshi taught that the path to reality is methodless, his students are often obsessed with forcing their bodies into preconceived postures.
>
> Two pure forms of teaching presence applied to therapy and education can be found in the work of Carl Rogers and

Charlotte Selver. Both have taught that the only goal of the therapist is being there for what is. Difficulties in transmitting their genius reveal how hard it is to comprehend presence. To be truly present with another person, I must find what interests me, what distracts me from my busy inner world, which is flooded with chatter and images. Rogers was fascinated by listening. The kind of listening that does not leave us feeling restless.

Have you ever made the mistake of trying to talk to certain "friends" when you are in distress? Here are some examples of unhelpful responses I have received: Me: "Yeah, I have been dealing with some anxiety since buying a house." My "fix-it" friend: "You bought in the wrong neighborhood. Here's my realtor's card; she'll find you exactly the house you're looking for." Or Me: "Yeah, I have been dealing with some anxiety since buying a house." My "story telling" friend: "I know exactly what you mean. When we bought our first house I didn't sleep for weeks—I mean, all those papers you have to sign! All that money! Of course, then we only paid $50,000, and today you couldn't touch that house for under $200,000. And did you see yesterday's real estate ads?" Or Me: "Yeah I have been dealing with some anxiety since buying the house." My "I can top that" friend: "I cannot even find an apartment to rent, much less buy. I wish I had your problem. You should feel lucky you are not in my shoes."

> -§-
> You can seed your partner's emotional clouds with empathy and help create a quick, refreshing shower of self-sharing.
> -§-

When I hear these responses, I do start feeling differently. Now I feel anxious and guilty. My Inner Therapist responds this way: "Maybe this has something to do with finally cutting the umbilical cord that has been keeping you trapped in the womb tomb of your narcissism." Thanks, Mr. Therapist, now I can sleep at night knowing what is wrong with me. My Inner Herbalist says: "Maybe you need to increase your zinc intake." My Financial Advisor: "It is not logical that you would have anxiety now. You have never been in better financial shape." There—that made the anxiety go away. I just told it that it was illogical and it went away…. Not!

What might an empathic response sound like? Empathic friend: "Are you feeling scared about whether you will always be able to make the payments?" And this is said not as a formula but with genuine interest and presence.

When someone empathizes with your chaos, it allows you to hear your confusion and thereby separate from it. You no longer are your confusion, but you are the observer of your confusion. This detachment from the confusion allows you to see it from another perspective. Even the word "confusion" suggests the problem. Con means "with" and fusion is of course a "merging with." So the problem with confusion is how to become "unmerged with" the situation.

A technology that I have found helpful in developing my empathic skills is Dr. Eugene Gendlin's "Focusing." One of the techniques used is to have someone guide you in focusing on what is really going on inside you. When overwhelming confusion is discovered inside, it is recommended that the guide not simply hear or echo back that overwhelm or confusion. It is recommended that the guide say something like, "A part of you is overwhelmed and confused." This helps the person being guided to take their head out of the bucket of soup and simply smell the soup from above it. From this vantage point it is easier to get a sense of what it is all about without being lost in it. It is as though you were lost in one of those mazes used to test the memory of laboratory rats, and someone picked you up above all the walls and corridors. You would then be above the maze and see it from a broader perspective. You could better understand where you were in the larger scheme of things, and how to take a more direct route to where you want to go. You might experience the relief of a-maze-ment.

> -§-
> Man invented language out of a deep need to complain.
> —Lily Tomlin
> -§-

Apologizing Is Not Empathizing

One reason I hesitate to say to someone "I am sorry" or "I apologize" is that it might be interpreted as admitting that I have done something wrong. There is no simple concept of "wrong" in a nonviolent consciousness. A consciousness of nonviolence leaves the idea of wrong (and therefore punishment) up to God.

Besides, apologizing is too easy. It is an indulgence in a feeling of guilt and can contribute to the avoidance of the deeper mourning—the soul's remorse, which is needed to develop true insight and therefore lasting behavior change. Suggesting I did something wrong is judging myself. If the other person was also judging me as having done something wrong, apologizing can reinforce that self-judgment. To the degree the judgment is reinforced, it will take longer for both people to release the pain that was stimulated and reestablish connection with each other. The longer the other carries the judgment, the longer they suffer with anger and resentment. The longer I carry the self-judgment, the longer it will take me to develop true insight into my behavior, which could give me the awareness needed for

-§-
The empathy softens the person up but the honesty causes the shift from stuckness. Empathy is the massage; honesty is the chiropractic adjustment.
-§-

true change. The sooner someone can come out of their head-full of judgments and into their body, the sooner they can begin the healing and releasing of the pain. Reinforcing the judgments through self-recriminating apologies serves to continue the re-wounding of the psyche and prevent learning and healing.

Apologizing can also plant a seed of judgment that was not there previously.

I cannot really have empathy for the other's pain until I feel the very real remorse that is repressed underneath any guilt I may have. I also need to have a compassionate nonjudgmental understanding of the feelings and needs that led me to do any regretful behavior. Staying in the guilt, saying I am sorry, thinking I did something wrong, thinking I am a jerk, and generally getting down on myself, prevents me from feeling the more painful remorse. And until I feel this remorse, I cannot offer the sweet salve of empathy to assist the hurting other in their healing process.

American culture is based on the idea of *retributive* justice, and therefore, we tend to beat up on ourselves when we think we did something wrong. This cuts us off from the compassionate power of *restorative* justice, which helps restore the hurt party's sense of well-being. It is this special quality of empathy called *compassion* that creates emotional, spiritual and even physical healing. Jesus channeled it when he healed the sick, casting out the "demons," which I believe were thought patterns of self-judgment. His holy act of empathic acceptance helped sufferers integrate their own unacceptable shadow parts, returning them to health and wholeness. Or to use more esoteric spiritual terms, it allowed them to shatter the illusion of their separateness from Source and remember their innocence. This channeling of divine healing energy has a long earthly history.

Speaking of the divine: someone told me that angels cannot give empathy because they are in constant bliss and cannot really connect with human suffering. That's why they envy us humans because we can give the healing gift of empathy to each other. Angels can only give love.

If I give empathy to make another feel better, it may be anxiety cloaked as empathy. While it is very likely that the other person will feel better, to be high-quality empathy, all my attention needs to be on their experience, not on thoughts of helping them. When the other starts to share their pain or joy with me, I would like to lose myself the way I do in a good novel. I read the novel not to help the author feel better, but to become one with the story for a while. The person must first feel the "presence" before the words of "empathy" are offered.

Sharpening the "Skill Saw" of Empathy

I find myself ever sharpening my skills at this mystical and profound art and science of empathy. The process of developing my skills requires that I use them with myself. When I am anxious or disappointed, I empathize with myself, feel my own sadness about that. Then I empathize with what made me chose to do it the ineffective way I did. Next I look for how I may have achieved the result I wanted. Life always provides me with another opportunity to practice again, having learned something more.

Groups have given me ample opportunities to sharpen my saw. Here's a dialogue that erupted after we were fifteen minutes into an introductory class on Nonviolent Communication.

Storm: "Why do you listen and pay attention to the men in the group, but ignore and criticize the women?"

Me: "Could you tell me what I did that you are calling ignoring and criticizing so I can tell you what was going on in me at that time?"

Storm: "See, there you go again, picking apart everything I am saying. It is just semantics and I am not going to play your stupid word games!"

After a long negotiation and much assistance from others, we agreed that the exchange would have gone much better if it had sounded like this:

Storm: "Why do you listen and pay attention to the men in the group but ignore and criticize the women?"

Me: "Are you hurt and angry because you're needing men and women to be treated equally?"

Storm: "Yes."

Storm needed empathy. And both of us needed a needs-based heart connection, so that she would be less likely to be fearful if I asked her to tell me what behavior she is calling "ignore and criticize." Without this empathic connection, it was no wonder that she responded as she did when asked for the observation. Also empathy on my part would have decreased the likelihood that the request for the observation would sound like "Do you have any proof, any evidence whatsoever Mr. Fung that you did not hallucinate the entire event?!" (This in not meant in any way to offend, slander, or even vaguely refer to Attorney for O. J. Simpson, Barry Scheck.)

When someone's pain has been triggered by me, if I can offer empathy to them before I ask, "What did I do?" it often reassures them that I do care about their pain, and that I am not just in defensive mode. This will increase the chances that they will continue to disclose themselves to me. Example:

Joe Blow: "You know, Kelly, you are not exactly the most conscious person on the planet."

Me (hopefully): "Are you frustrated about wanting more sensitivity to your feelings in this situation?"

Another way I try to help the other sense that I am really trying to be understanding is to empathetically guess what someone is reacting to or observing. Example:

Joe Blow: "That was certainly critical of you."

Me: "Was it when I said to Sheila that I was frustrated and wanted connection with her need for sharing the story?"

Here I am trying to empathize with the observation rather than just ask "What did I say that you are calling a criticism?" In my experience trying to guess the observation is usually interpreted as sincere interest, more so than asking, "What are you calling a criticism?" or "What are you reacting to?" or "What is your observation?"

Empathy Before Explanations

Empathy is spiritually protected and cannot be misused. The intention of empathy is to connect, not to direct or correct, and explanations before empathy sound like excuses. Example: Jane (in an angry tone): "Why are you late?" John (in an anxious tone): "Well, there was this big accident on Eighth Street, right where it intersects with Mission Drive, near where the old Wal-Mart used to be. And I thought about pulling over and giving you a call but then I would be even later."

Each word digs John in deeper. And it is painful for Jane to be pretending to listen, too. She is waiting her turn, which makes her a good waiter and therefore a lousy listener. Waiting dilutes listening and the lack of listening presence is always felt on some level. She will likely be getting more and more resentful as she thinks "I am the victim here and now I have to listen to all his excuses?" Empathize with the other's misperception before you offer them your correction. An example of this might be: Jane: "You are totally irresponsible. How could you have forgotten again to lock the door?" John: "Yes I hear how frustrating that is for you. However it was Ed who left it unlocked this time."

You can have technical skills at empathy and still have low octane presence in the empathy.

"Why's" Aren't Wise

Don't use "Why...?" when trying to empathize. It is wise to use no "Why's." "Why...?" Questions take the other person to their head and out of their present feelings. A better question might be: "Are you (or "It sounds like you are) feeling _____ because you _____?" "Why" is a cognitive, mental question that leads one to start thinking and explaining. When I am empathizing with someone's feelings, I support them in staying in their feelings as long as they need to. When someone has painful feelings and is asked a "Why...?" question, it is frequently interpreted as an attack. As children, we were traumatized by angry adults asking angry "Why...?" questions. They were on a fault-finding mission, gathering evidence so the prosecution could convict, sentence and punish us.

-§-
The difference between a healer and a fixer is that one empathizes until what is needed emerges and the other assumes what is needed and goes about giving it whether it is wanted or not.
-§-

If someone is hurting or in fear, the "Why...?" question can sound like you are saying that they should not be feeling what they are feeling. The "Why...?" question can be heard as questioning or invalidating the person's feelings instead of validating them. Example: Lonely Husband: "Gosh I miss my wife." Unhelpful Friend trying to be supportive: "Why don't you join a dating service?" When the lonely husband hears this, he misses his wife even more; she at least used to listen to him sometimes. Or: Nervous Traveler: "I am scared to fly in airplanes." Unhelpful Friend trying to be supportive: "Why do you think planes are not safe?" Unless the nervous traveler has great confidence in himself, he is likely to start doubting and berating himself: "My friend is right. I should not be scared of flying. What's wrong with me?"

"Why...?" questions are particularly distracting from the healing process when they take the conversation down a track different from the one the person in pain needs to explore. Grieving son: "I feel like I can't go on since my mother died." Anxious Friend: "Why can't they put more money into cancer research?"

Here the friend is really expressing their own pain and anxiety, which is likely to distract the son from his grieving process. The son may end up answering the question or trying to be there for his anxious friend's pain—at the expense of his own process.

Don't bring in any of your own theories. Don't lead the witness by saying "Is this a secret longing to be your father's wife?" This falls under the category of asking "Interesting Questions," which reveal more about the questioner's theories and less about the person being asked. Better to ask "Interested Questions," where the intention is to show interest in and focus on the person being questioned. I also avoid informational or historical questions like, "How old were you when you started to feel this way?" or, "Does anyone else in your family have a history of depression?"

Connecting Before Correcting

How important is it to connect before you correct? Here's a funny example of the consequences of not connecting first.

There were two motorcyclists who were getting cold as the wind blew through the zippers in the front of their jackets as they rode. They decided to turn their jackets around and zip them up the back. As they went on down the road they hit a rock and went flying into the ditch. A nice chiropractor came by in his car, saw what had happened and got out to help. A paramedic finally arrived and said, "What a shame, they are both dead." "Yeah," said the chiropractor, "I did what I could. When I arrived they were both breathing, but their necks looked terribly twisted so I gave them a major adjustment."

Human Needs Behind All Inhuman Deeds

A major block to developing empathy for others and wholeness within the individual is the fear of receiving empathy. It is particularly tough for men to receive empathy, since they have had gender role training to stay in their heads with the "hard" superior, masculine, dominator emotions like anger, contempt, and disgust, instead of ever feeling the "soft" inferior, feminine, submissive emotions like fear, hurt, or sadness. Boys are taught they are "sissies" or "effeminate" and should feel ashamed, as it is "inappropriate" for boys to cry or be scared. The macho motto is "Don't cry. Get mad, then get even." In a dominator society, such as ours, the men prepare for war, or at least the war of the workplace, which requires that they never give in to the "soft" emotions such as caring, compassion or empathy. How are they going to win the war if they care for their competition? It is a little easier for women to give and receive empathy since their gender role includes caring for crying children by comforting them (a form of empathy).

Here are two more fears people have about receiving empathy. One is that they will lose control of themselves, fall apart or go crazy. Another is the fear that if they open up to their painful feelings, they will cry forever, or be stuck in the pain forever. This fear cuts people in half, keeping a wall between their heads and their bodies. In other ways our culture supports this form of schizophrenia by teaching us to believe that people deserve to be punished, and that we really are, in a static sense, wrong or bad if we have done certain things. This not only prevents sanity within individuals, but blocks the clearing and release of painful beliefs that keep people separate.

An example of this is a young mother, Stacy, who came to me with her father, Maury, seeking to resolve her incest issues before they destroyed her marriage. It was very tough going because of the father's fear of self-empathy or compassion. Maury was totally willing to acknowledge what he had done to his daughter and all too willing to condemn himself for it.

Why do I say, "all too willing"? Because Maury's willingness to condemn himself generated great guilt and shame within himself, which completely blocked him from having true empathy for his daughter. It also blocked him from going deep into, and sharing, his own pain and sorrow about what he had done. This sharing was something his daughter was spiritually very hungry for. It was easier for Maury to stay up in his head, blaming himself for what a monster he was, than to feel into the enormous sorrow of his daughter's devastation. Each time his daughter would begin to get in touch with her pain and express some of it, he would unconsciously interrupt her with an apology.

Stacy: "Daddy, I was so hurt, I just wanted you to love me so much that..."

Maury, interrupting her mid-sentence: "I am so sorry sweetheart. I cannot believe how stupid and selfish I was." Each time this happened Stacy would stuff her pain and try to take care of her father's pain by reassuring him.

I tried to empathize with the father's guilt and shame that was preventing him from really hearing his daughter, but each time he would block me by going up to his head and defending his righteous self-condemnation.

Maury: "No, I do not deserve any compassion, after what I did to her I do not even deserve to live." (In the background of my head I can hear a chorus of my right wing conservative friends saying "At least you got that right!") It was hard work to get him to see that right there and then his daughter needed him, and once again he was not available because it was too scary for him to let go of his righteous self-image as a cretin. The jackals were screaming so loud in his own head that he was unable to hear his daughter's pain, which was exactly what was going on years ago that allowed him to molest her in the first place. He had been so caught up in his own anger, hurt, emptiness, and shame that he had no empathy for his little girl's fear, confusion and hurt at the time of the incest. Once again

-§-
A person can not forgive themselves until they have mourned what they did.
-§-

146

she needed his parental presence, and he was off to Siberia on a guilt trip. I tried to offer guidance

Me: "Can you understand the forces at work that made you do what you did?"

Maury: "Sure, I was a totally selfish sick individual, who apparently hated himself so much he wanted to take it out on other individuals."

Me: "Too easy. Not deep enough. What were you feeling and needing that led you to choose to have sex with your daughter?"

Maury (in tears): "I was desperate for relief from self-hate, and loneliness, and I wanted to feel loved."

Me: "I understand you hate what you did. Can you just understand what made you do it?"

Maury: "No, I cannot go there. I cannot forgive myself! If I forgive myself I might do something like that again."

Me: "So it is real scary to let yourself feel acceptance of your loneliness and need to be loved and connected with?"

Maury: "Yes."

Me: "It was the lack of acceptance of that feeling and those needs that led to your acting them out in the first place. Also if you do not feel and release that pain you will not be able to be present to help your daughter let go of her pain."

"Okay," he said with a sigh and a "whoosh" of an exhale like a dying man's last breath. With that he dropped down into his body and expressed the inconsolable sobs of a completely forlorn man. After twenty minutes he raised his head and said "I am ready."

"Ready for what?" asked Stacy.

"I am finally ready to really hear your pain," said this new man.

"Oh, Daddy, I have missed you so much!" cried Stacy.

"I have never been able to believe or understand that you could feel that way after what I have done. I have heard you say that before, but for some reason that I do not understand, I completely trust what you're saying. And all I can feel is grateful that you care about me at all and so very sad that my guilt stopped me from hearing you up till now," said Maury.

"And, Daddy, what you did has destroyed my life, my self-esteem, and all my relationships up till now," said Stacy.

With some coaching from me, Maury was able to reflect back Stacy's pain from his heart: "You have felt a horrible confusion in your life and shame about yourself, and this has created the loss of all your relationships so far."

"Yes, I have thought all my life that there was something really wrong with me that I would let such a thing happen. And then when you pulled away it just confirmed that I was worthless," said Stacy.

"So all your life you have felt this kind of shame and core defectiveness, and when I pulled away you felt all the more worthless," said Maury.

"Yes," said Stacy with a sigh of relief, "And I just need to know how you feel hearing all this."

"Oh, Sweetie, I would do anything to take your pain away," said Maury.

"Then tell me what you are feeling deep inside right now," said Stacy.

Maury started to say something quickly but then stopped himself. Slowly he closed his eyes and just sat there. Then his stomach began to quiver, his chest went into a heaving convulsion, and his head started to go up and down as the sobs poured from deep in his throat and abdomen. At first Stacy sat silent and shocked. Then her body became animated, her eyes refilled with tears, and she reached out to wrap her father in her arms. No verbal answer was ever given to her question about how her father was feeling. No verbal answer needed. The knowing and the understanding was so thick in the room, any words would have diluted the deluge.

A lifetime's anguish about incest is not likely to be cured in a single therapy session. This was a huge first step for Stacy and Maury in their journey toward wholeness, but the real work lies in the aftercare.

What allowed the transformation to occur was the healing potency of presence. If I had only had conventional psychotherapy techniques to use, I am doubtful much would have happened. Virginia Satir used to tell me, "It's not the technology, it is the technician." A big part of what allowed this technician to offer potent presence was that I had earlier allowed myself to receive major empathy for my own pain at being abused as a child.

The End of Empathy

We all know people who cycle around and around in their story of having been abused. Even if they get to their feelings and receive empathy for them, they feel compelled to keep telling their story. They also keep acting their story out until they allow the empathy to make them conscious of their ongoing unmet needs. If an adult lost a parent in early childhood, they may need to grieve, but at some point they also need to get conscious that they still need mothering or fathering, and go out and find it. As I work with clients in therapy, there comes a point when empathy no longer serves them. So even though, as the great psychologist and author Rollo May said, "All healing begins with empathy," it does not end there. May also explained that empathy is like massage, but honesty is the chiropractic that makes the fundamental structural adjustments in someone's belief systems, attitudes and life.

I once had as a client, an eighty-year-old women, who had literally been in all kinds of therapy for forty-five years. She could write books on her various neuroses, from an Adlerian or Freudian or Gestalt or Behavioral or Cognitive or Transactional or Rogerian perspective. She would cycle through her different theories with me—until I started to give her my honesty. When I did she became furious and insisted that I give her empathy instead. To which I replied, "I feel uneasy about continuing to give you empathy when I think honesty would be more helpful to you. I wonder if that irritates the heck out of you." She told me that she hated me, fired me, and I have not seen her since. I like to fantasize that I cured her from her addiction to therapists.

Empathy When You Can, Honesty When You Can't

One time not to empathize is when the request for empathy is sensed as a demand. By demand I mean that the person asking for the empathy is going to withdraw, get hurt, angry, judgmental, or punish you if you do not empathize. In these cases it's better to give honesty, silence or use protective force (such as walking away, hanging up, or filing a restraining order). Example: Jane to Dick: "It really hurt me when you went over to talk to Jill instead of me."

Dick senses that Jane is going to get angry at him if he does not empathize. So Dick might say: "I feel irritated right now. I am trying to unhook myself from taking on responsibility and guilt for your hurt. Would you be willing to talk to me about this tomorrow?"

-§-
The key to empathy with others is empathy to self.
-§-

Any time I am "supposed to" give empathy, I hate the experience and I will not do it. You cannot give presence, love, empathy from "supposed to" energy. It just does not work, any more than I can get "turned on" because you put a gun to my head. Nor can other people give you empathy because they should, just because they are your friends. You simply can't give empathy from "should" energy.

Empathy In the Extreme

As long as you are hating yourself, you cannot let in empathy. Without self-empathy you cannot stop seeing yourself as weak, stupid, or lazy. As soon as you let the empathy in, you can forgive yourself and, like a caterpillar, come out of the cocoon of self-hate and judgment, see yourself differently, and then start to act differently.

Empathy can work wonders even for teenagers, and even in extremely violent situations. I used to be a counselor in an adolescent treatment center. One day, two young gang members, one African American, one Latino, ran from the Offender Treatment Facility to escape the restraining arms of the staff. The only thing in their minds was their intense hatred for each other and an overwhelming passion-ate urge to beat each other to a pulp.

Once they got into the open space of the basketball court they indulged themselves in their orgy of hate. One gouged the other's eyes. The other swung wild haymakers in an attempt to knock the head off his nemesis.

JR, my Vietnamese coworker, and I each grabbed one of the com-batants and dragged them to opposite ends of the facility. I took my wounded warrior into my counseling office and locked the door behind me.

Me: "Whoa, dude, looks like you're going ballistic."

Him: "You got that right!"

Me: "He must have really done something intense. You do not usually just go off on anyone."

Him: "Yeah, man, he's been trying to steal my stuff while I am at school and he's been trying to snake [steal] my girl."

Me: "So I guess you want him to know that you are not going to take that lying down."

Him: "Yeah man, I ain't no chump."

Me: "And you would like him to know just how angry you were?"

Him: "Yeah, man. That's what I was doing before you stopped me."

Me: "Yeah, well I wasn't enjoying how you were letting him know that. You know we have a difference of opinion about what is the best way to express feelings."

-§-
Sometimes trying to be sensitive is the most insensi-tive thing you can do.
-§-

Him: "Yeah, I know, say the feelings, make requests, but he's a real punk, treating me like a friend just so he can dis [disrespect] me when I'm not looking."

Me: "So you are really angry because you wanted to be respected for the trust you showed him. You let him be your friend and introduced him to your girlfriend, and you wanted him to respect that by leaving your stuff and girlfriend alone."

Him: "Yeah, man. We were bro's."

Me: "So are you feeling hurt because you really like him and wanted to stay friends?"

Him: "Yeah, but I never keep friends, something always happens like this."

Me: "Are you just feeling hopeless about ever having friends you can count on?"

Him: "I never had nobody I could count on."

Me: "Sounds like you are sad because you really would have like some people in your life you could count on and who would respect you."

Him: "Yeah, man, but we got to stop this now.

Me: "How come?"

Him: "Because how am I going to be able to beat him up when I am starting to feel all calm and shit?"

Empathy Eases and Expands

One day Mataya, then one year old, was fussing. Her cries wafted through the house. I felt tense and stressed. My partner Deb reminded me that Mataya was teething. I then felt a relaxing shift in my body, as compassion for my sweet little one's pain flowed through me. It is a high and holy practice of holistic selfishness to maintain an expanded consciousness of empathic understanding for everyone. Why do I call it selfish? Because I benefit by feeling more connected and less tense in the face of events that used to annoy me. (Like babies crying in airplanes on take off and landing. As I understood they were crying because the change in pressure hurt their ears, my pain and irritation decreased.)

-§-
If you are hearing whining, you are listening with a closed heart. Open your heart, and you will hear fear and pain mixed together.
-§-

I flashed forward twenty years in my imagination. I pretended that I was remembering what it was like to have a baby's cry blessing my daily life, her tiny soul, her sweet innocent spirit sharing her vulnerability with me. I remembered its honeysuckle sweetness, I tasted the preciousness of the sound. It is her. She is sharing herself without withholding, without restraint. I pray I can always hear the purity of her reaching out to me, and be touched in the same way. When her cries turn into whining words, when she screams at me in anger and frustration, please, dear heart of mine, remember this connection between our souls. The form has changed but the truth of her being reaching out for comfort remains the same. Could I, would I, listen with the same compassionate ear to all such cries for connection — whether they be in angry words, polite excuses, put-downs, or punishments. If only I could hear what their mothers heard once upon a time, "Oh, my child needs me. How blessed I am to be able to respond."

-§-
All communication is either an SOS or a care package, a please or a thank you, a need or an offering to meet a need.
-§-

Chapter

THE DANGER OF DESERVE

My family taught me that I do not deserve anything. So now when I want something, I hear a voice that says, "I am greedy and don't deserve it, " leaving me with feelings of shame and depression. My New Age friends tell me I do deserve everything, so then I think, "Well, if I deserve everything, why don't I have it? It's not fair!" This leaves me feeling angry and bitter. Thanks, guys, now I have two belief barriers to overcome in order to allow success or love into my life.

Belief number one is "I deserve it." This belief makes me mad and jealous when I see that little know-nothing twerp Deepak Chopra, splashed all over TV and Oprah, and those obnoxious pictures of his mansion overlooking the ocean just a couple miles and a universe away from my house in San Diego. (Just kidding. Deepak Chopra has been very kind to me, allowing me to do presentations at his Center, etc. He has also been super supportive of Nonviolent Communication, calling it "the missing piece" in his own work. Thinking, "I do deserve" can stimulate anger. Why? Because if you do deserve something, you should have it, right? "Should" thinking makes us angry and is a form of denial of reality, because it says that "what is" should not be.

Belief number two is, "I don't deserve it." This belief leads me to depression and poor-me helplessness. The fear that I do not deserve starts to come up whenever someone tries to give me something I want. It sometimes leads me to deflect or block the gift in some way.

I want to go beyond "deserve" to "I want..." or "I choose to have...." If we bring into our consciousness the concept of "deserve," then we also bring in the concept of "do not deserve." Thinking "I do not deserve" can stimulate feelings of shame, guilt or fear. I want to receive abundantly not because "I deserve," but because I want something and choose to give it to myself. I choose not to go up into my head to debate and theosophically theorize about whether I deserve something or not.

To say that someone deserves x, y or z implies that they have done something "to deserve." For example, if you say to someone, "You deserve abundance," the implication is that they merit abundance because they have paid their dues. What about the idea that "it rains on the just and the unjust," the deserving and the undeserving? In Alfie Kohn's great book *Punished By Rewards*, he questions the marketplace foundation of our Western sense of justice: "To assume that fairness always requires that people should get what they 'earn' — that the law of the marketplace is the same thing as justice — is a very dubious proposition indeed." He goes on to explain how looking at personal relations in terms of the marketplace deteriorates and depersonalizes personal relations.

What about the possibility that abundance is there for the taking? Certainly this would make more sense to the eye because if you look around, you sometimes see violent people with disgusting values that have lots more fame, fortune and family than the "good,"so-called deserving people. We project onto the universe the experience of our families, where the rule often was, "You knock on the door of being given to through obedience." We believe there is conditionality to the universe, just as there was in our families. We have trouble imagining that the universe is unconditionally giving to us. We think we have to deserve, or at least believe we deserve, before we will receive.

It is a fun New Age religious trap to believe, "As soon as I can believe I deserve, I will receive. If I am not receiving as much as I want, it's proof that I believe I don't deserve." It's easy to get stuck in this "wheel of misfortune." Maybe the universe is waiting for you to let go of the idea of "deserve" and "don't deserve" so you can be open to receiving. What if you could get tired of wrestling with whether you deserve or not and be humble enough to acknowledge you do not know? What if you could acknowledge that you just want x, y or z, whether you think you deserve it or not? Maybe then you could take responsibility for choosing it or not.

The Envy Exercise

I have been stuck in the stage of thinking, "Look at that teacher or workshop leader, look at the crowds they are drawing. Their stuff is not nearly as good as mine. They do not deserve that kind of recognition." Jealousy and hurt about others getting more than they deserve contributes to a kind of moral righteous superiority. "At least I am not getting more than I deserve."

Nobody keeps track of your "deserve score" anyway. So it doesn't really matter to the universe whether you get more or less than your idea of what you deserve. But it does make a big, big difference in what you are willing to ask for. If you are feeling jealous of anyone in this world, it is probably because you are not asking fully for what you want. I recommend doing the following exercise: Write down the names of the people you envy, and what they have that you envy. Then write down the essential elements of what they have that you already have, clarifying what needs these elements fulfill. And finally write down what steps you might take to get you more of what you want and when you plan to take those steps.

-§-
Judgment and analysis of others are dissociated expressions of our own wants.
-§-

Here is one of mine:

Person: Stan Dale, Director of the Human Awareness Institute, author, teacher.

What does he have that I envy? A large community of loving people to interact with, teach and care for.

What needs are fulfilled by these things? Community, a niche, a way to contribute, affection, emotional and intellectual stimulation.

In what ways am I already meeting these needs? I have a growing community of loving people. I present workshops that help meet my need to contribute.

What steps might I take to add to my abundance? I can finish and promote this book. I can collaborate with the Human Awareness Institute and The Center for Partnership Studies in my city.

When will I do these things? I will finish the book by June 30th, and promote it for the next two years. I will call the key people in both these organizations and ask how I might help their work in my area, before September 1st.

It is important that I intentionally set a date for completion to help bring the action into reality.

The Dream of the Field of Diamonds

I once dreamed that there is a field of diamonds with different kinds of people in it. There are those who are scared, with voracious appetites for diamonds. They pick up and hoard hundreds of diamonds, desperately trying, but never succeeding, to fill the holes in their souls. There are those who are like little children, never questioning whether they deserve the diamonds or not, but simply surrendering to their own natural fascination with the sparkling rocks. They pick them up, put some in their pockets, and share others with their child-like friends in a fearless celebration of the wonder of the world. Then there are those who are intrigued by the wonder of the stones, but can't find the flexibility to bend over, to humbly reach down to pick up the diamonds. Still other people do nothing, forever wondering what they should do.

Then there are those who ponder whether they deserve these stones or not. They are caught in the paralysis of philosophical analysis. They are scared to receive without first thinking they deserve or have somehow earned the right to receive. In one of her songs, Ruth Bebermeyer sums it up:

> I like being aware that there's nothing to achieve.
> Life's a gift I have only to receive.

Chapter

THE MYTH OF MOTIVATION:
APPLYING COMPASSION INSTEAD OF COERCION

Everything I do with the intention of motivating myself back-fires. Within the intention to motivate myself there lies an implicit "should," which immediately sets me at odds with myself, and frequently triggers rebellion.

Human souls come into this world full of passion and purpose. And then well-meaning parents and teachers start trying to motivate them. Rosemarie Anderson, author and social commentator said, "Who would have thought that play could be turned into work by rewarding people for doing what they like to do?" Did you ever have to motivate yourself to go to recess or play your favorite game? Do you now have to motivate yourself to hike your favorite trail, read your favorite book or have sex? I hope not.

Speaking of sex, there are people who have to, excuse the pun, pump themselves up psychologically to have sex. It has become an obligation that they feel duty-bound to perform. It is a sad state of affairs, and perhaps the cause of many affairs, that something as alive and profound as erotic energy can become as lifeless and mundane as study hall used to be. It comes from a basic distrust of human nature, expressed in the concept of Original Sin. In our Western culture, there is a great distrust that human beings will do what is needed unless they are threatened with punishment or coerced with rewards.

I wish there was more understanding that it is the very use of coercion, positive or negative, that breaks or deadens the spirit, which is the source of motivation. This is not only true between people, but within oneself. So the more I try to motivate myself to do whatever I think I "should" do, the less energy I have to do it.

Educational geniuses, people who have Ph.D.s and head our educational institutions, are forever coming up with new methods to coerce children into doing what would otherwise be intrinsically satisfying. I am reminded of the pizza-for-books program in Georgia called "Book It." This is where teachers give out coupons, good for a free pizza, for every 5 books a child reads. This was sponsored by that bastion of altruism Pizza Hut. And of course the children then picked the thinnest books with the biggest print. Why? So they could get past that nasty hurdle called reading as quickly as possible, to get to that which is really valued, the goodie, the pizza. The net result is a bunch of fat kids with eating disorders who hate to read.

-§-
No one in a relationship can take the other person's power. We can only give our power away to each other.
-§-

Right now my 4½ year old absolutely loves books. She has her own book shelves, and asks me to read to her several times a day. I need to be sure to keep her away from American schools though, or she may start responding the way most kids in our pop culture do when asked if they like books: "yuk!!!"

Then there is our old buddy Representative Newt Gingrich. He spoke at my alma mater, the University of West Georgia, to praise the education department for paying third graders two dollars for each book they read. His motto was "Adults are motivated by money, why not kids?" I start to wonder, "What's wrong with me?" I never got paid to read. I used to read because it was fun. Maybe I got ripped off. Maybe I could get together with a bunch of other baby boomers that were abused in this way and file a huge class action suit against the federal government. We could get billions in back pay.

Every afternoon in the summer, when there was no school, I used to climb a stile over a barbed wire fence, and walk through tall fennel weeds, to get to Dave's house. Dave's house was a shack on my Uncle Jake's property. It had once been occupied by a caretaker named Dave who had succeeded in drinking himself to death. Long abandoned, it still had a small, creaky porch with a cot on it, just right for reading and napping. I could not wait to get a few hundred yards away from my Aunt's stern eye and shaking finger, her never-ending avalanche of anxiety, worrying and complaining. Dave's house was an escape. Once there, I could travel several centuries and thousands of miles away, as I joined the Mongol hordes. I could read about the heroic passions of *The Golden Hawks of Genghis Khan*. I could find a way to my own grief through *Greyfriars Bobby*, a story about a Scotch Terrier. When his master died, he dug his paws raw trying to get under the cemetery wall. Whether I was feeling grief or grandiose, each entry into that world of books was an adventure in aliveness. I was not made or asked, or bribed, or rewarded to read; I was allowed.

Organizational development expert Douglas McGregor says that the answer to the question "How do you motivate people?" is, "You don't." We can motivate ourselves and others to do things through threat of punishment or promise of reward, but at the cost of our passion. And it is this passion to do something that gives us the energy to produce excellence. It is like a father teaching his child to ride a bike. Which is more important: The child learning to ride a bike quickly? Or the father and child maintaining and developing a rich, loving connection? How tragic that so many children are afraid of their father's anger or disappointment. If we focus on maintaining a high quality of relationship between the two, then they create learning together. The child can learn how to learn, and how to ride a bike. The father can learn how to teach in a way that enriches his relationship with his child.

This is the relationship I want with myself as I enter new realms of creativity and self-expression. I never want to achieve, learn or create at the expense of a kind, gentle, loving, supportive relationship with myself. It is so easy to fall into trying to coerce myself. I know of many a father who either cracks the whip, or begs and pleads with his child to become a great bicycle rider. I know many individuals who cruelly coerce themselves to achieve and develop in certain areas. And they do gain mastery or achievement in an arena. In that sense, coercion can work. But at what cost to our relationships with our inner child and selves?

As I write this, my first book, I am challenged to practice what I am preaching. Moment by moment, I am choosing to monitor whether I am either threatening myself with a harsh stick, or holding out the carrot of extrinsic reward. Do you know where that image comes from? It is from an old cartoon; a carrot hangs in front of a dumb animal and behind the animal is man with a big stick about to hit the animal. What kind of animal is between the carrot and the stick? A jackass!

I have been an abusive father with myself, and now I am often afraid of me. Most of my effort to teach or motivate myself has been of the "cracker or the smacker" variety. All too often it has either been the cracker (Brit-speak for "cookie") of an extrinsic reward—money, sex, acknowledgment, or simply the relief from self-hate and depression. Or just as likely, it has been the smacker, beating myself up with a barrage of self-hating actions ranging from simple self-derision or vindictive criticism, to complex compulsions like alcohol/drugs/food, relationship roulette, schoolaholism, guru submission, depression, accident proneness, exposure to danger, illnesses, boredom, and suicide attempts. As with any abusive relationship, it will take time to change my patterns and redevelop trust. I am reminded of the last lines of a song that Dr. Rosenberg wrote for his son Brett. It is written from the perspective of the son, speaking to his father about their relationship.

> And even if you should change your style
> It'll take me a little while
> Before I can forgive and forget.

> Because it seemed to me that you
> Didn't see me as human too,
> Not till all your standards were met.

I need liberation from the concept of self-motivation. As long as I am trying to motivate myself, I am caught in a Catch-22. I am schizoid: there is one me that is trying to motivate another me. I feel a sense of endless futile struggle, as I keep one foot on the gas pedal and the other on the brake. I make little progress because I am just as rebellious as I am coercive.

Why do I even have to motivate myself? Do I have to motivate myself to have sex, play my guitar, or play my favorite game, basketball? No, because I am connected with the intrinsic reward for doing these things. Did it take hours of focused, strenuous effort to get to an enjoyable level of mastery at these things? Of course. Did it take delayed gratification and discipline? That was not my inner phenomenological experience. If it had been, I probably would have rebelled and not been able to focus enough to develop any skill.

Because I was raised by religious Calvinistic joy- and life-haters, the idea of delaying gratification triggers my fear that we are talking repression. I much prefer the concept of "maximizing my pleasure through strategic timing." I do not want to think in terms of delaying my gratification, but rather strategically planning to have it when it will have the maximum impact. A small example would be having a wonderful meal in a restaurant and getting close to being full. I like to stop before I get full and bring the rest home in a container, not because I am delaying gratification but because it will taste so much better in several hours when I am really hungry again.

-§-
I do want to move toward my goal, but not at the expense of my soul.
-§-

Someone once asked J. Krishnamurti, the Indian sage described by the Dalai Lama as "one of the greatest thinkers of the age," if there was a difference between self-discipline and suppression. He said that the only difference was that self-discipline is a more subtle form of suppression and repression. He went on to say that the mind that is really intelligent is free of self-discipline. He said,

So you must observe, become aware how your own thought, how your own feelings are functioning, without wanting to guide them in any particular direction. First of all, before you guide them, find out how they are functioning. Before you try to change and alter thought and feeling, find out the manner of their working, and you will see that they are continually adjusting themselves within the limitations established by that point fixed by desire and the fulfillment of that desire. In awareness there is no discipline.

Like Krishnamurti, I want to move beyond self-discipline into enlightened selfishness.

I love to play basketball. I love the endorphin rush that total immersion into the timelessness of the moment brings, and the release of physical and emotional tension that comes from a hard workout. I can maximize all these effects if I do a few hours of writing before I play. The contrast between the sedentary activity of writing and the physical endurance required on the court is sublime. My pleasure is increased by the sense of satisfaction that comes from excelling at my sport.

Five Steps to Elan Vital

The concept of self-motivation stimulates images of struggle and inner conflict. I prefer something more like self-liberation, where I am liberating the trapped energy of the wild child that lives within. As a kid I never had to motivate myself to go out and play. There is a powerful creative and productive urge within me, and I need only to get out of its way. I choose to create an environment that makes it easy to love what I am doing. Here are five steps to getting out of the way of your own elan vital, your vital creative energy:

Step 1: Self-Empathy

I frequently have an inner jackal god that commands me to "get busy." When I try to appease this god by making sacrifices of my time, or making myself do something that I think would meet its standard of productivity, I give my power to it and submit to its oppression. I then start to lose motivation to do anything. I find myself strangely compelled to sing "Working On a Chain Gang" under my breath as I drag one leg behind me through my day. What actually needs to happen is to give empathy to that "get busy" jackal. If you could get inside my head you would hear this conversation:

Jackal: "What the hell are you doing? Get busy. Do something. You are wasting your life!"

Wise Giraffe: "I sense fear, anxiety, and old hurt around a need to be fully engaged in the joy of full, creative self-expression. I sense a request to dive headlong into the middle of the rushing river of life. I also hear the fear of self-contempt, and a need for a gentle accepting relationship with self."

Step 2: Quit Rewarding Yourself

When I started to write this book, I told myself I would buy myself a new car when I finished it. It took me months to figure out why it was so difficult to make much progress. The wild wonderchild of my creativity did not want to be bought and sold, and was unwilling to help me with my project. Give yourself stuff because you want it and need it, not because you have earned it or deserve it. Care for the many sides of your Self, and creativity will follow, instead of trying to be productive so that you will earn your self-acceptance. Creative writing teacher Julia Cameron recommends we give ourselves "artist dates" where we go out and romance and indulge ourselves in an experience of creative rejuvenation. This would include things like going to an art gallery, a walk in a Japanese garden, or—for me—a long talk with my zany writer friends, like Diana Loomans.

Step 3: Interrupt All Comparison Thoughts

Comparison thoughts are ideas like, "Why am I just now getting my first book written when that little sissy wimp John Gray has twenty best-selling books out there?" (Just kidding John. I actually admire your courageous heart after seeing you actually working live with people. And you were very generous to take the time to read my book and write me an endorsement—all at no charge, of course.) Or a woman might think, "I know people tell me I look nice, but I am nothing compared to someone with real beauty."

Psychologist Dan Greenburg wrote a book called *How To Make Yourself Miserable*. One of the most "powerful and ingenious techniques" he recommends for "achieving misery" is comparing ourselves to others. He has drawings of the faces of a "normal" man and woman with little centimeter numbers inscribed on them. You are directed to measure your face (or the face of your prospective lovemate), compare your measurements to these Olympic specimens, and then meditate on the difference. He reminds us that any variation, no matter how slight, is a defect. And if you find no differences, you are referred to the section on How to Make Yourself Miserable if You are a Beautiful Person.

We all know beauty is only skin deep and that the measure of your worth comes from your soul's expression in life. For this Greenburg offers his Aid to Evaluating Your Accomplishments. It is a picture of what Greenburg calls four ordinary people who were chosen at random. The first one is a twenty-six-year-old patent office clerk, A. Einstein, who formulated a theory about relativity. What theories have you formulated? Then, Greenburg offers us a youthful piano player, W. A. Mozart, who composed his first symphony and three sets of sonatas by age eight. List your compositions by age eight. Next is Prince Abdullah al-Salim of Kuwait, who receives a salary of $7,280,000 weekly. What's your salary? I recommend that as soon as you recognize a thought as being of the comparison variety, pull it out like a weed, because if you do not it will multiply. Here's two ways to pull it out.

1. Let it remind you that whatever you are jealous of or compare yourself to is a shadowy expression of your dream for yourself. Take the time to write out what that desire or dream is, and then strategize how to move towards it. For example, I was jealous of, and comparing myself to, author John Gray. So now I am writing this book

2. Stop the thought. Just refuse to keep thinking it. Tell yourself, "I have been there, done that and I am choosing to spend my energy

on other things." Then focus your attention into some medium like reading, writing, or conversation. If the thought is persistent, you can get a "God Can." Write out the thought and put it in the can. Whenever the thought comes again tell yourself "Nope, I put that one in the God Can and God can take care of it for me."

Here's a poem I wrote to help you recognize and understand your own Comparison Jackals:

The Comparison Jackal
by Kelly Bryson

Jackals are creatures that live in my head.
And whenever they speak I start feeling dread.
There are many breeds, from Critic to Poor Me,
Forever diagnosing what is wrong with me.

They are Comparison Jackals all ten feet tall,
Pointing out to me that I am relatively small.

They remind me I am nobody, not famous like Amos.
It is not something I am proud of, in fact I feel shamous.
That I haven't done more with the gifts I have been given.
I have hardly done nothing. I have hardly been livin'.

And I do not have much money, not one share of stock.
On Christmas I will betcha I get rocks in my sock.

Now I am not much to look at, with a growing pot belly.
And it's hard to be macho with a girl's name like Kelly.

Now Comparison Jackals are a fast-breeding lot.
They never get tired of pointing out what you are not.
Even if you've won an Olympic gold medal
Will your Jackal be happy and finally settle?
No, it will scream "What's the matter with you?
If you'd only tried harder you could have won two!"
So whether you try your least or your most,

You can trust your Jackal to move the goal post.

So how do you win the comparison game?
You are going to lose if to win is your aim.

You must lose to win, which is simply done
By refusing to play games that aren't fun.
To lose the fear to appear second rate
And be uniquely you is a new kind of great.
To lose yourself into selfless esteem
And think your own thoughts and dream your own dream.
And always to ask for 100 percent
Of what ever you want so you'll never resent.
That way you'll never miss out on a chance
To invite yourself to enter life's dance.

Please consider doing the following exercise as a way of becoming more conscious of your comparison jackals. Just becoming conscious of them can help you deal with them in a more powerful way, because what you are conscious of, you can have some control over. What you are unconscious of, controls you.

What are your comparison jackals? To help flush them out, complete the following sentences:

1.   The problem with me is I am too _____.

2.   The problem with me is I am not _____ enough.

Step 4: Create Collaborative Community

The great psychologist Alfred Adler identified the need for significance and belonging as the primary psychological drives for pack animals known as humans. These needs can be met so much better in the community of a workgroup—which energizes the individual, creates synergy, and thereby increases output. I enjoy serious working for only an hour or two before I start to feel sluggish. However, I can play all day. I can play all night too if I have other people to play with me. I have noticed that when I go by myself to play basketball, I really only enjoy practicing my shooting for a few minutes. If someone comes and we can shoot together or play one-on-one, I may last an hour. But as more and more people come, we sustain each other in an energy field that can soar for hours.

In case you already have too much motivation, here are some exhausting games you can play to depress yourself.

Exhausting Game #1: Fritz Perls, the father of Gestalt Therapy, articulated the Top Dog/Underdog model of motivation. Top Dog says, "You should do your paperwork." Underdog whimpers back, "Yea, but I do not feel like it," or growls, "You cannot make me!" First figure out what your number one "should" is like. It might be, "I should do my taxes early." Then you spend hours going back and forth, with Top Dog demanding action from yourself, and Underdog whining and making excuses for not doing it. If you work hard and dedicate yourself to this dialogue, you will soon be too exhausted to do your taxes, which will give you the perfect excuse not to. This will confirm what Fritz Perls says: "Underdog always wins."

-§-
If you are thinking you "should" get something done, You've made a choice that will not lead to fun.
-§-

Exhausting Game #2: Screw up all your discipline and make yourself do those things you have been avoiding. You will then need several days to recover from the energy drain. The product, whatever you create from this kind of motivation, is low quality. Again it is similar to having one foot on the brake of your car and one on the gas — and then stepping hard on the gas. You will get somewhere but it will cost you. That is how I got through a four-year undergraduate college program in just under thirteen years.

Maybe Life *Is* a Box of Chocolate

If a friend gives you a big, beautiful box of chocolates, you have at least two choices about how you will receive them. One choice is to receive them hesitantly, with fears of not showing the proper amount of appreciation. You might start eating them with an attitude of guilt. "Oh, I should eat these to show my appreciation." Or you can choose an attitude of "Yippee, Chocolates!" I think life is like the giver of that box of chocolates, and would probably prefer that they be received with an attitude of enjoyment not drudgery.

Before I open my box of chocolates (otherwise known as my life) in the morning, I want to make sure I remember how to receive. I need to remember what it was like before I learned about the concepts of sin, of being bad, and of not deserving. I need to remember what it was like when I was aware that everything was being given to me as a gift. This was before I started taking credit (or blame) for everything.

I remember being only four years old, waking up just as the first rays of light slipped through the window of our house in the aptly-named Valley of the Sun. I would sneak out of our house using a technique my sister taught me called "Indian feet." That is where you put the toes and ball of your foot down before you put down the heel, to make less noise. Once outside, I would hop on my little red scooter and take off through the suburban streets of Phoenix, Arizona. I was bursting with joy, excitement, and adventure. "Who's up?" I would be thinking. "Who wants to play with me?" I just knew that everyone wanted to see me and play with me.

I would roll up to the first house where I saw or heard any signs of life and simply present myself. "Hi, I am Kelly. I live down the street. What are you doing?" And often the answer would be "Well, we are fixing breakfast." "I haven't eaten yet, what are you having?" I would inquire. And of course my innocent self-invitation worked like magic. No, it was magic. When I had finished my wonder-filled waffles, I would be off to the next house. And the next house. It was a terrific way to start my day, just to present myself and let people nurture me. I think of this time as my Garden of Eden days. It was like when Adam and Eve lived in Paradise, and they did not have to work or do anything. All they needed to do was enjoy the garden, eat and play.

Then they learned about concepts like "good" and "bad." This enabled them to be doing one thing and thinking they should be doing another. This was the beginning of the fall. After this they had to toil in the soil, otherwise known as getting a job. (If Maynard G. Krebes, the sixties freeloading beatnik from the TV show "Dobbie Gillis" had been in the Garden, he would have been screaming "EEEEEKKK!!!! Do not say that word 'work' around me. You know I am allergic to the 'work' word!") Before I do anything I want to remember that I can choose to remember that I am still in paradise, that there is nothing I should do or have to do. I can choose to just start opening up the chocolates *de' jour*.

There is a part of me that wants to see progress, the sweet fulfilling feeling of accomplishment and creative pride. Another part of me just enjoys the process of creation. I also enjoy the effect of creation on my being. Sometimes when writing or talking, I discover and clarify an understanding that than becomes a new part of my consciousness. There is also the joy of being swept away on the currents of creativity's river. Sometimes when I first put my little raft in the relatively calm waters of the river's side eddies, my pen to paper, or fingers to the keyboard, it can almost feel like effort. But as I push my way further into the river, the strength of the current kicks in. Then I must simply hang on and keep up with where I am being taken.

-§-
"All real life is in the meeting," says Martin Buber. The quickest way of contacting God is through a certain quality of meeting with other people.
-§-

I am afraid that even holding out the carrot of "a satisfying sense of accomplishment" is an attempt to coerce myself in the same way all my teachers and parents did. It begins to create a split within myself. I have never had to give myself a pep talk to get me to load up all my fishing gear, drive all the way up the mountain, and climb through the bushes to go fishing. I have friends who are rock climbers. They do not have to tell themselves, "Think of how beautiful it will be once you get to the top." They know that beauty is awaiting them, but if they held it out like a carrot and tried to motivate themselves with it in the same coercive fashion their parents and teachers used, they would resist. Even if they did coerce themselves to climb one mountain, the next one would feel like all the more work. So I want to be very careful about forcing myself to do something that I might potentially love doing. Instead I want to remember that I live in paradise, where each day is a gift, and work is play.

Getting Paid to Play

Work is not an activity. It is an attitude. An attitude based on fear and scarcity. When people think they "have to" work for a living, it is partly because they were taught as children that "there are many things you have to do whether you want to or not." This sets people up to be not conscious of other, more joyful, more life-serving possibilities. I like the axiom, "If there is a want there is a way." So if you want to play and still receive pay, there is certainly a way. But in order to believe this you will need to give up two sacred beliefs. One is that suffering is necessary and noble. And two, that we live in a limited, scarce, dog-eat-dog world.

Those who truly play at what they love contribute the most to themselves and the world. Mother Teresa played nurturing mother to the world. Albert Einstein loved to play with numbers and theories. Jonas Salk enjoyed playing doctor, and Jesus played compassionate spiritual father. Remember what he said when the disciples rebuked the little children for running up and jumping on him? Something like, "Suffer the little children to come unto me, for such is the Kingdom of Heaven."

Everything I do with the intention of motivating myself, backfires. Just within the intention to motivate myself there lies an implicit "should." Motivating myself tells my subconscious that I am not motivated. Even if I put up little pieces of paper on the wall, with phrases to remind me of the reasons why I want to do certain projects, it does not help.

For example, I put up notes on the wall about what writing this book would do for me: "Writing the book will provide me with more ways to connect with more people," and "It will help me discover more of myself," and "It will provide insights and tools to help people relieve their suffering." If I am coming from the self-conflicted attitude of trying to motivate myself, my Top Dog mind says, "Yea, you're right. I really should be doing something to connect with more people and provide tools and knowledge to relieve their suffering. And God knows I could use more insight into myself, so maybe I should be a little more motivated." Each well-intentioned, inspirational nudge becomes the image of my Aunt Willie, shaking her finger at me, saying, "You're not going to get any supper unless you finish your homework!" The nudge becomes a nag.

Now that I have discovered that I actually love to write, I need to be a little careful not to make myself sick of it again. One way I made myself sick of it was by forcing it down my throat when I was in college and graduate school. It is just like with food. If you love butter pecan ice cream, as I do, two surefire ways to make yourself sick of it are to force it down your throat when you're not hungry, and to make yourself eat too much of it. When we are coerced by rewards and punishment we lose awareness of what we really love and how much of it we really want to imbibe.

I was at the pediatrician's office when my daughter was six days old. There was a nutrition poster in the doctor's office giving new parents basic advice about how and what to feed their children. It said, "Never make you child eat anything, because first of all you cannot, and secondly it will damage their ability to notice when and how hungry they are." This is what happened to me with respect to my creativity and productivity. I was coerced by rewards and punishment to the point that I was no longer connected to my own need to be creatively productive. Sometimes now, when I get a little taste of my own creativity, I notice how delicious it is and how starved I am, and I pig out. This leaves me with a bad taste in my mouth and makes me doubt that I really enjoy creating at all. It restimulates the original allergic reaction that teachers and schools created to my creative expression in the first place.

I cannot write when I make myself write. Especially I cannot write about how we free ourselves from coercive forces. I simply journal until the Top Dog merges with the resistant Underdog. Then playful productivity emerges. These two parts of me are just two needs that require a way to cooperate. One need is for a satisfaction, another is to have fun. Someone once said that they wake up every morning torn between two wonderful urges. One is to enjoy the world and the other is to contribute to it. May we always trust that there is a way to do both, even at the same time.

The transition from inertia to movement is often the phase that takes the most energy, and includes the most pain. I once asked Thom Hartmann, Ph.D. award-winning, best-selling author of *The Last Hours of Ancient Sunlight,* "What does it take to actually finish writing a book?" His answer was "It is similar to picking blackberries. Sometimes you just stick your hands into the thorny bushes and grab them even though you know you are going to get all bloody. If you notice that you have been staring at those blackberries a long time, suffering from the fear of getting all bloody, the compassionate thing to do may be to run screaming into the blackberry bushes."

From Oppressed To Oppressor

When we are externally motivated, coerced by reward and punishment, we lose touch with why we might hate to do something. We lose touch with our own needs. We have been like rats in a Skinner box experiment. We have our learned behavior — pulling the lever to get the positive reinforcement — which include acts like being cooperative, pleasing our boss, or taking care of our spouse. But we lost connection with our instincts to forage for food, to nest, and other activities that would nourish our whole being.

-§-
I reject motivation,
And instead choose
inspiration,
Sending my mind
on a vacation
To a more playful
paradigm!
-§-

One of the treatments for alcoholics is called "antibuse." Antibuse makes alcoholics feel sick if they taste alcohol. Sometimes I feel as if I was given a large dose of anti-productivity-creativity-dream. Whenever I make an effort to fulfill my dreams, doing something creative that is not directly linked to a reward like money for survival, I start to feel that old familiar sickening fear arise. My culture and schooling, with its use of reward and punishment, effectively crippled my autonomy, my entrepreneurial spirit, and any intrinsic motivation to create. For many years my spirit was so broken and confused that all I could do was work in the factories that need docile, subservient, externally motivated robots.

I even became "institutionalized" myself. That is, I became one of the spirit/autonomy breakers for hire, when I went to work for adolescent treatment centers. "Treatment Center" is an ironic name. As if these adolescents kids had developed tuberculosis and had to be sent away to be cured. Most of them were there because they hated how they were treated at school and home. Most were there because they had more spunk and smarts than their more obedient and cooperative peers. My job, which I hated, was to get the little tykes to do what their teachers and parents told them to do. We used techniques like stars and candy bars for rewards. We used punishments like solitary confinement, increasing the quantity of medication, and not letting kids see their families — all in an attempt to coerce them into attending their boring classes in their dehumanizing schools. All the while, the therapists, social workers and administrators were constantly reassuring each other that they were doing it all "for the good of the kids."

-§-
It is the process, not the product or project, that counts.
-§-

From time to time I get invitations to train the staff of similar institutions. Decades after my own tenure, I see staff still using the same inhumane strategies mentioned above and other techniques of reward and punishment that I believe severely damage the psyches of these teens. I am glad there is something new I can offer.

Craving Creativity

If one drinks in only inspiration and never expresses out in the form of creation, there is no flow. Keeping creativity flowing is similar to breathing: after inspiration comes "expiration," the act of creating externally. I can spark inspiration by exposing myself to the creative expression of others, people who are on fire with the same passion I have. If I am writing, I can read inspired writers, who inspire me in turn. Embers from their fire sparks my soul. And then I want to let that spark set fire to my soul's work, keeping my eye on the vital essence of my vision, as my soul takes one step at a time down the path of my passion. Breathing in, breathing out. In with inspiring art, scenery, music, oratory; expressing out with poems, songs, books, letters. In with great sex, out with great sex. In with provocative movies, out with written screenplays. In with soulful speakers, out with soulful speech. In with soul food, out with creative cookery for all my friends. In with powerful musical, theater, dance, comedy, sports performances — out with the same. So many intoxicants to imbibe, so much disorderly, crazy behavior to express.

The idea that manifestation is 1% inspiration and 99% perspiration depresses my inner child and blocks him from creating. If your creation is taking 99% perspiration, it stinks and you need more inspiration. With more inspiration, more breathing in of life, you can let spirit do the work. Find a balance between inspiration and perspiration. If you're stuck on at a ratio of less than fifty-fifty, then you need more inspiration. We do not need motivation, we need inspiration. If we get inspiration, then motivation will follow. Neither writing nor creating is miserable. Thinking I *should* write or create is miserable.

There is a difference between documenting moments of clarity about what I want to create in my life, and trying to make myself do what I think I should. If the intention is to remind myself of a moment of inspiration I had about what would be fun to create, that's wonderful. If I take the moment of inspiration and try to turn it into a cattle prod, woe is me. I really am longing for a return to the experience of work as a voyage of discovery, like the books I used to read about the adventures of Silver Chief — a very loyal, intelligent German Shepherd dog.

We are born with the innate ability to enter that magical world of adventure and creativity, the imagination, and if we are stifled we yearn for it. Like the child who watches other children on the playground from the window of the detention hall, the soul aches to create. If the soul, torn between the security of obedience and the freedom of flight, stays obedient to internalized authorities, it slips into the self-motivation maze.

I chose to make a compassionate relationship with me my first priority and achieving outer goals second. Many times it is the greatest act of compassion for myself to strive with great drive and passion towards some goal. It is an act of self-hate to be forcing myself to keep working out of fear. I need to listen to myself and my body to know the difference. I want to quit forcing myself to fulfill an agenda. I want the agenda to be developing a caring, loving, nurturing, accepting connection with me and then to take action. You must give up "must," and learn to trust if you're going to motivate yourself compassionately. Psychologist Albert Ellis told us that we must quit "musturbating."

Static Stinking Thinking

Static thinking is a great way to damn up the river of creative and productive expression. You can chant incantations (or "I-can't-ations") until you hypnotize yourself into a zombie like-trance: "I can't seem to get inspired," or, "I can't afford to buy a computer," or "I can't find the right people to work with," and so on, ad infinitum. If you chant these incantations over and over, the power of belief will paint you into a very small corner of your consciousness.

A funny example of this is when I am looking in the refrigerator, screaming at Deb, "I can not find the mayo!" She patiently responds, "It is right in the front shelf."

"I can't find it!" I say in earnest, hoping she will come and find it for me. The problem is that if I do start to see the mayo that is sitting right in front of me, I have to make a liar out of myself. So my subconscious mind protects me from that humiliating event by making the mayo invisible to me. The mind has great power to create blind spots in order to protect itself from fear or shame.

Another type of static thinking is "have to's" and "had to's." This includes things like, "I have to work eighty hours a week just to make ends meet, so I can't learn to play the piano." Here's one I love: "I have to stay home and take care of the dogs, so I can't really take vacations."

As I experiment with my life, and my mind and body, I find that there are no "have to's" and "I can't's." What truly exists is, "I am scared," or "I'm confused about how to." For example, I used to think, "I can't afford to buy a house." Then I translated that into, "I am confused about how to buy a house."

I expressed this out loud to a few people. They turned me on to this awesome concept called a mortgage, where a bank puts up the money. I would still be renting if I had not made the translation in thinking. Martin Luther King, Jr. observed that, in oppressive cultures, governments will sometimes let people think, the government is bad, but are afraid to allow them to take action to change anything. The same is true within my own inner jackal government. It is okay to say "I am lazy" but my ego freaks out when I start to take action.

One big fear that keeps me from starting or finishing a project is the fear that I won't be "good enough." A little motto that helps me with that is, "Anything worth doing is worth doing poorly." Or its corollary, "Anything worth doing is worth regretting later." These will free up your creativity better than the motto: "You can not fall out of bed if you sleep on the floor." One very successful computer software company has this as its guiding motto: "Fail often, succeed sooner."

Why is it that when you do not feel like doing anything you have way more time on your hands than you want? Then when you really feel like doing lots and lots of different things, you haven't nearly as much time as you want? If you quit trying to get yourself to produce, you can start to let yourself create. In mythological terms we need to return to Eden and leave the Paradise-Lost hell of work and toil. My Uncle Jake used to explain, "Them cows need to give their milk or they get sick." Maybe people would find more cow-like contentment if they could find the balance between giving their gift, and grazing in the green grass of whatever restores their soul's energy.

How did we enter this coercive relationship with ourselves? Dr. Rosenberg once told me that if a culture can convince its members of the following three things, they will become good slaves of the culture:

1. There are some things you have to do whether you like to or not.

2. There are people called "authorities," who will tell you what these things are.

3. If these authorities punish you for disobeying, it is for your own good.

I choose to use my creativity, humor, talents, skills, resources and wisdom as a way to help evolve a new culture. I believe this is an exciting, satisfying possibility for many of us. I believe it is totally possible for us to do this in a way that follows our bliss. Whether we choose to paint or park cars, cook or write a book, if we can do whatever brings us the most fun and satisfaction, with a consciousness of contribution, we will have the joy of sacred pleasure and the gratitude of sacred service.

Re-Sourcing: Connecting With Source

When I am scared and telling myself that I am not seeing enough progress, I have found yet another way to procrastinate. That is like hanging my head after I miss a shot at basketball instead of noticing that I shot the ball short and to the left, and begin making the correction to my shot. Do you know which baseball player holds the record for the most strike outs in history? Babe Ruth! So instead of indulging in the self-pitying notion that I am not seeing the progress I should, I ask myself: "How can I feel more energy to move toward my goals?" Some answers:

1. I can talk to people who are excited about similar goals.

2. I can talk to people who are interested and enthusiastic about my dreams.

3. I can sit down and draw a picture of what it would look like to achieve a certain goal.

4. I can write a short paragraph and pretend it is a newspaper announcement about my achieving a goal. The emotional body does not know the difference between role-play and reality. Pretending can give you an appetizer taste of the feeling of accomplishment even before you achieve it.

5. I can ask other people to support me or collaborate with me in achieving my goals.

6. I can take some guilt-free rest.

7. I can indulge in some energy-generating recreation to recharge my battery for creation.

8. I can imagine I am at my own funeral, listening to an eulogy celebrating all the specific contributions, achievements, and creations I accomplished.

9. What connects you to your passion and purpose? Choose your favorites from among the following activities: Writing, dancing, reading, telling or listening to stories, nonfiction books, seeing movies, meditation, walks in nature or in the city, conversation with certain creative friends. How about fishing, watching babies feed, feeding ducks, playing with babies, calling old friends, surfing the web, talking to counselors or psychics, repotting plants, planning the future, meeting with mastermind groups, writing science fiction short stories, writing poetry, philosophy, making love with an older or newer relationship, brainstorming, painting, playing music, singing, cooking, swimming, riding a bike, throwing a Frisbee, walking a dog, riding a horse, flying a kite, eating sushi, reading scripture, taking a sauna, chanting, yoga, climbing to the top of a tall palm tree. Which direction is your own personal land of milk and honey?

Chapter

COMPASSION UNDER FIRE—
HOT TALK IN HOT SPOTS

One of the most selfish and satisfying experiences of my life has been teaching Nonviolent Communication in war-torn areas of the world, where it is most needed and wanted. I have had the opportunity to do this in the Balkans, Northern Ireland, as well as in Israel and the occupied territories of Palestine.

I had been longing to go to the Balkans since my friend, Dr. Nada Savic, Director of Psychology at the University of Belgrade, had called me in desperation. The Bosnian war was raging, and Nada explained that she was in great personal pain as the ravages of war surrounded her. She felt helpless to stop her own country's Serbian army as they raped tens of thousands of women and children in a calculated military strategy to punish and scare people into obedience. She felt overwhelmed by the magnitude of the need for healing, conflict resolution, and peacemaking education among her colleagues and in the refugee camps. However, she was connected to a very large network of teachers and psychologists throughout the Balkans and was determined to expose them to the Nonviolent Communication process. There was a great and growing need for healing and understanding if the recurring cycle of ethnic hatred and violence were ever going to be laid to rest.

I, too, felt a deep pain and a need to respond to the horrors occurring not only in the Balkans but in Northern Ireland, and in the Middle East. A part of my pain and frustration was that although I had the desire to contribute, I did not have the financial resources to go to these regions and provide my services.

I was in the middle of processing this pain internally when I was invited to speak at a large festival called the Whole Being Weekend in Julian, California. About four hundred and fifty people attend this festival each year. For the last sixteen years, I have taught Nonviolent Communication there. I was in the middle of facilitating a workshop at the festival when this pain started bubbling up and I expressed it verbally. This was probably inappropriate—according to the standards of most professional mental health schools of thought—but I come from a different school, where teachers and therapists are appreciated for their humanness and vulnerability. I began to cry and explain the pain I was in, knowing what was going on in Serbia, and how much I wanted to do something about it. A white-haired old gentleman asked, "What's stopping you?"

"Money," I replied. "The people there do not have the money to fly me over there, although they have volunteered to take care of me once I get there." The old man asked me to talk to him after the workshop.

After the workshop the old man approached me and asked me how much I needed. I told him and then he disappeared for a while. The next time I saw him he approached me with a check in his hands and tears in his eyes. He explained, "Ever since I heard about the systematic rape of women and children going on over there, I too have been in a lot of pain. I have been desperately needing to do something that could help. I thought of sending money to the Red Cross or something, but I worry it is not going to really help things change. Thank you, thank you for giving me a way to help that I trust will help." And with that he gave me a check for the full amount of what I needed to make my trip. At first I felt my usual resistance to receiving. Jackal thoughts said, "You do not deserve this," "He should not have done this for you," and "You manipulated this man with your tears." However, I could truly feel the relief it was bringing him to have me receive his contribution, and how painful it would have been for him had I refused. There was a quality in that exchange that I pray for in all of my giving and receiving.

So thanks to Rev. George Whitford, for that was his name, I was off to Europe and the Middle East to respond to the invitations I had received from Nada, and other centers for Nonviolent Communication.

From the Ire of the Irish to Peaceful Protestants and Compassionate Catholics

"Granny talk, that's all you talk!" yelled the burly Irish Catholic priest to the Protestant ex-nun turned feminist.

"See — that's the very kind of patriarchal put-down I would expect from someone like you. You invalidate my age, sex and emotions all in one phrase," she volleyed back.

I was at my first stop on the trip, Northern Ireland. I was facilitating a workshop for Protestants and Catholics, courtesy of the international Center for Nonviolent Communication. The workshop was being held at Correymeala, a huge compound and community of about 3,000 people dedicated to healing the conflict in that religion. Besides the general public, some of the Correymeala staff were invited, and the workshop was followed by three days with the staff of the Irish and also the British centers for Nonviolent Communication.

Believe it or not, the above exchange was a big relief after two-and-a-half days of "Nicey Nice Talk." (My experience of the Irish was one of particular politeness.) Author Scott Peck calls it "pseudo-mutuality," when everyone talks about the importance of peace as an idea but no one reveals what is going on inside themselves from the neck down. There is an unconscious taboo against talking about what feelings are going on between the people right now in the present.

After two days of polite cooperation, totally devoid of any life, emotion, or controversy, I began to feel a great fear, and painful emptiness, welling up in my stomach. I spent the whole night tossing and turning unable to sleep with my Jackals screaming, "Who the hell do you think you are, pretending to be some big-wig international conflict resolution expert. What a joke. You are going to screw everything up for Dr. Rosenberg and the Center for NVC."

Another whiny voice said, "Please, I just want to be a humble counselor. Let me go back to San Diego and live a simple life."

But it was too late. I was thousands of miles away from home with forty-something ever-so-polite Irish citizens. I was face-to-face with a most dreaded realization: I was going to have to practice what I preach—argh! I might have to ask someone for empathy and understanding for this horrible pain, instead of maintaining my nice, professional veneer, playing the role of the all-tolerant mediator. Meanwhile I was seething with judgmental thoughts about what freaking phonies these Irish are. I was faced with having to withdraw my projection, which was, "These Irish people are a bunch of polite phonies" and remember that Dr. Rosenberg said: "All labels are the tragic expression of pain and unmet needs." My pain was coming from my unmet need for an authentic connection at the emotional level with these people. I was the one that needed to quit being polite and professional and start being transparent, and true to what was real inside me.

I came to the workshop the next morning filled with dread and anguish, and looked around like a lost pup for any possibility of comfort. Then an angel appeared. Rachel, the wife of the director of the facility, asked if I was okay, and if she could get me some tea. This is something some Irish women do every hour, on the hour. I said, "No. I am not okay. I am in HELL!"

The next fifteen minutes or so are a blur. All I remember are Rachel's beautiful, slightly teary eyes, soaking in all my anguish about not knowing how to get the peace process progressing in the group, my fear that everyone wanted to leave, and sadness that my dream was turning into a nightmare. She gave me perfect understanding and empathy for all my pain and fear. I felt the healing energy of empathy coming through very powerfully. What touched me the most was her pure, sweet intention to connect with and comfort me.

I shared my pain and tears in front of the entire group of workshop participants. Most reacted with shock, fear or amazement. However, it did seem to open up the space and provide permission to express the ugly, dark and painful emotions. This was when the Protestant ex-nun-turned-feminist began sharing her anger, hurt and sorrow about how she had been treated by priests in her church. Although it was not directed at the Catholic priest in our group, it triggered him to express his pain in his native tongue of "Jackal Language" by calling what she was sharing "Granny Talk."

All hell broke loose between the Catholic priest and the ex-nun. Other participants were drawn in. It looked as though we were all headed for World War III when the priest did a complete about-face. He demonstrated that he had not been sleeping through the previous two days of sessions. He said to the ex-nun, "I am hearing that you are very angry at the way men in authority have used their power and that you want respect for your way of expressing yourself."

"Why, yes," she said, with surprise, "but every time I open my mouth or try to contribute something, someone like you comes along to invalidate it."

The priest responded, "It must be very painful to need appreciation for your contribution and never get it."

Woman: "Yes, when I was a nun, I started several wonderful programs to help people. Then some patriarchal ass would come along and cancel it without giving me a chance to be heard. And if I tried to be heard, I was labeled a troublemaker."

The Catholic priest responded, "So what I said reminds you of all the years of doing your best to make a contribution to people, and then some male authority comes along and changes it, leaving you feeling just devastated. And then you have to face the anger about not getting heard about the devastation."

"Yes! Yes," says the ex-nun. Torrents of tears start to flow.

The priest turns to me and says, "It works. I cannot believe it, but it works. All my life I thought I had to fight strong women, but now I can see that all I need to do is give them empathy. I cannot believe how simple it is, and how I've missed out all these years, especially with my family."

For the next two days these two people were inseparable, spending all their free time and lunch times together, just absorbing all they had to show each other of their shadow sides. You could almost see the exchange of wholeness going on between these polar opposites, Catholic Macho Man and Protestant Feminist Woman. This initial dialogue opened up a flood of feelings and healings around the issues of male/female relations, in-groups and out-groups, us and them. This is at the core of the Protestant/Catholic conflict.

One Protestant young man, Tim, sobbed as he told how he was ostracized when he refused to talk badly about his Catholic friend, even being beaten up by his schoolmates for being a Catholic-lover. Not only did he get the releasing, relieving elixir of empathy to his feelings of shame and hurt, but we also got him to explore and understand what forces were at work in his perpetrators. Other young men in the group had participated in such scapegoating activities and were suffering from shame and guilt about it. We learned that their behavior was because of their fear that the scary finger of accusation would next be turned toward them. It was this fear that led them to participate in the scapegoating and beating of Protestants.

-§-
"There is always a human need behind every horrible deed."
-§-

When Tim finally realized at a deep emotional level that the very human need for safety lay behind the beatings, he was transformed. Understanding the human need behind the horrible deed turned his hate into compassion.

Other participants said that most Irish children on both sides of the conflict are put to bed each night with descriptions of those awful Catholics (or Protestants) who killed their family members, and how they should demonstrate their love for Mommy and Daddy by getting revenge. When anyone begins to sympathize in the slightest way with the other side, it triggers all this hate and desire to prove their love for their family through violent revenge.

After these breakthroughs, the work went deep, with many insights, much healing and skillbuilding. Both the British and the Irish Centers for Nonviolent Communication sent trainers to Northern Ireland to take training with me. They have since written me that the workshops deepened their skills and helped them grow their bond with each other. Many new people have begun practicing Nonviolent Communication in both countries. I continue to get e-mails about how these skills have changed the lives of the people who learned them.

Battle in the Balkans

By ferry and train, I made my way to Zagreb, Croatia. I started with a half-day workshop. The participants were a mixture of Nongovernmental Organization (NGO) workers, members of the feminist movement, and members of the Croatian Anti-War Campaign. Many of these people, I later found out, were in deep conflict with each other and afraid for political reasons to be vulnerable in front of each other. I connected with people working at the refugee camps, and teachers working at junior colleges. Workshops were arranged at the refugee camp and for the junior college students and staff. The refugee kids were delightful, playing with me, singing songs in English, and allowing me to teach them "Giraffe Language." They loved the Jackal and Giraffe puppets I used to teach them NVC. One ten-year-old boy named Vlade shared about how the kids called him "Fatso." We all gave him empathy, and then role-played how he might deal with that judgment using Nonviolent Communication. I used the puppets to help Vlade articulate his feelings and get the other children to hear him.

First I took the Giraffe puppet and started to focus the other children's attention on Vlade's feelings.

Giraffe puppet to children: "I am sad when I hear what Vlade is telling me about being called "Fatso." I want us all to be cared for and treated with respect. How do you think Vlade was feeling when some of you were calling him "Fatso?"

Croatian girl: "Like we didn't want him around?"

Giraffe puppet: "Thank you. I really like that you are trying to imagine what Vlade might have been thinking. If he were thinking that you all did not want him around, how do you suppose he might have been feeling?"

A Croatian boy named Drozin: "Like nobody cares about him?"

Giraffe puppet: "Have you ever felt like nobody cares about you?"

Drozin: "Yes."

Giraffe puppet: "Were you sad or mad?"

Drozin: "Both!"

Giraffe puppet: "Yes, thank you. Many times I have two or three or four different feelings happening at the same time. Maybe Vlade was feeling both mad and sad after being called "Fatso." Would you be willing to ask him if that's true?"

Drozin: "Were you sad and mad, the other day when I called you 'Fatso?'"

Vlade (with a crack in his voice and a tear in his eye): "Yes, I was."

Giraffe puppet: "Thank you for hearing Vlade. Now I was wondering, Vlade, do you feel glad that he was able to hear you?"

Vlade: "Yes, but now I am scared that they are going to call me a little sissy girl for crying."

Giraffe puppet: "Hum, I see. Yes, I can see how that could be scary. Would you be willing to ask the other children how they are feeling about your crying and sharing your feelings with them?"

Vlade: "Okay. Is anybody thinking I am a sissy?"

Three or four of the children shake their heads or say, "No."

Drozin: "I am sad that I made you feel bad because I know what it's like to feel that nobody cares about you."

Giraffe puppet: "Thank you very much for sharing your feelings that way, it touched my heart. But now, Vlade, suppose instead of Drozin saying he was sad," (I pick up the Jackal puppet), "he had said something like: 'You are not just a sissy but a big, fat, Fatso sissy. Ha, ha, ha, ha, ha!'"

Vlade: "I would punch him in his big fat stupid face like I always do when I finally catch him."

Giraffe puppet: "I see. I am worried though that that has not been working too well for you. What if I showed you a little 'tongue fu' and see if that does not work better. Are you willing give that a try?"

Vlade: "Yeah, okay."

Jackal puppet: "Yeah, you are a big fat Fatso, sissy!"

Giraffe puppet: "Now don't respond right away. Just listen to all the Jackals that start going off in your head about how you are going to punch him in the face when you catch him, and how it's not fair, and how he is a mean, stupid kid. Then get into it and enjoy and feel all your feelings of rage, hurt, shame, and fear. Then, when the storm of these feelings passes, see if you can tune into what need he is trying to express through all these judgments of you. Remember names, labels and judgments are always sad expressions of unmet needs. And if it helps you focus in, you can use the magic question, the most powerful question in the world: 'Are you feeling _____ (and then guess what he might be feeling) because you want _____?' (and then guess what he might be wanting)."

Vlade then closed his eyes, breathing big breaths in and out. I was encouraged because I had not told him to breathe. He just figured out that this is what he needed to do to tame his inner jackals. He then opened his eyes slowly and said, "Are you afraid that all the kids might start picking on you, and you want them to keep picking on me instead?"

Giraffe puppet: "Go ahead and ask Drozin this question, okay?"

Vlade to Drozin: "Are you afraid that all the kids might start picking on you, and you want them to keep picking on me instead?"

Drozin: "I never thought about it but yes, I think that was true at first, but now I just really hate you."

Vlade: "Oh great, now he hates me. You are making things worse!"

Giraffe puppet; "Yep, Yep, I can see how you might start feeling angry toward me and scared because you were hoping to make things better between you guys. Sometimes though things have to get worse before they can get better. It is important sometimes to initiate conflict so you can bring out the anger or hate that is causing people to treat each other poorly. Also, I am pretty sure that that hate was in there before we started this conversation. I am excited now because I know it is inevitable that if we keep talking and listening to each other this way things will get better. Would you be willing to guess what he hates you for?"

Vlade: "What do you hate me for?"

Drozin: "Because you hit me hard, and besides if I am your friend no one will be my friend."

Vlade: "So if I quit hitting, you would you quit calling me 'Fatso'?"

Drozin: "Maybe, but I am still not going to be your friend."

Vlade: "That's okay because I know that if you hang out with someone who is not cool, then everyone will think you are not cool too."

Drozin: "Exactly. I can't believe you get it. That's cool!"

From this point I did not push them to make any agreements about stopping the name-calling or hitting, as I was concerned that they might rebel against the pressure. It also felt to me that there was a delicate opening and a sweet flow of connecting energy that would do its healing work between them, if allowed.

As I left the refugee camp I saw the two boys talking with each other. And although I could not understand what they were saying, because my translator was no longer present, my inner ten-year-old told me that they were speaking innocent little-boy talk about frogs, Frisbees and foolishness. Just what little boys should be talking about.

The next day my Croatian hosts took me to what looked like an American high school building. I was told that the grade level system in the schools in the Balkans is quite different from those in the U.S., but that this school was the equivalent of a junior college. The junior college students were interested in Nonviolent Communication, particularly in how it could be used to help them deal with one of their teachers whom they saw as particularly oppressive. The workshop went very well and I could see they were excited about "getting it." All except for the thirty-year-old school psychologist in attendance. He sat off to the side, wearing a proud, broad smirk of skepticism.

With unabashed amusement, just short of outright laughter, he asked if I actually believed that what I was teaching would work in the real world. I told him that it worked in my real world, but I could understand his doubt. Just then we were walking together toward the school's gymnasium. He chuckled and asked if I would like to try it on the school's basketball court just down the hall. Basketball is Croatia's national sport, and Croatians are proud of their dominant position in European basketball.

Basketball is also my favorite game. When growing up poor and isolated on the farm with my aunt and uncle, I played often. Basketball is one of the few sports you can practice by yourself without expensive equipment. A homemade ring of stiff wire nailed to a pine tree was my stadium. I learned to turn my loneliness into lay-ups, and my height disadvantage into hook shots. I desperately wanted to play high school basketball, but my aunt and uncle told me that the drive into town was too long. This not only failed to dampen my lifelong obsession with the sport, but fueled it.

I hid my glee at the psychologist's request behind my best poker face, and gave him a nonchalant nod of acceptance. I heard my own Mr. Macho Man inside me say, "Little do you know that you just challenged Zorro to a sword fight."

The duel began. I played the only style I was familiar with: "Heads-up, in-your-face, one-on-one, kick-ass basketball." The talented young Croatian was able to keep up with my style, making the games very close. Afterwards, however, he approached me and in his halting English said, "You don't play basketball like compassionate giraffe, you play more like fierce jackal." I had mixed feelings about hearing this. On the one hand I enjoyed his acknowledgment of the quality of my game, but felt disappointed that I had not conveyed what Nonviolent Communication is really about. I had tried to explain that the bigger part of com*passion* is *passion.* It is not about being nice, or passive, or giving in, but about being holistically selfish and compassionate with oneself first, sometimes in a very assertive way. To give in or give up on my needs is a form of violence to myself and my relationship with the other. I did my best to clear up this confusion with him but I could tell he did not totally get how we could be compassionate and self-assertive at the same time.

I did not make a convert out of the psychologist, although I did plant a few seeds of confusion. I felt much more hopeful about the students and the possibility that a new generation might see possibilities for peace through the power of passion with compassion. I was also grateful for the opportunity to show a model of standing up to someone without standing against them. I hoped it was meaningful to the students to hear someone question one of their authorities in a nonauthoritarian way.

From Croatia I took the train to Hungary and then down to Belgrade, Serbia. Because the Balkan War was in high gear with intense fighting along major roads, I could not take the highway that connects the two cities, the so-called "Highway of Brotherhood." Dr. Nada Savic had arranged an extensive agenda for me, including a trip to Montenegro to meet with a group of psychologists there. I took a plane from Belgrade to Kotor, Montenegro, the most beautiful city I have ever seen. On the Coast of the Adriatic, the ancient city's old town is partly surrounded by a moat. The hillside is dotted with remnants of castles past. And the people were delightful. They greeted me at Kotor's airport (a farmer's field) with an enormous trumpet lily, intuiting my need for beauty. We spent three days immersed in learning and a deep sharing of ourselves.

The workshop was held in an ancient, ivy-covered church building, right on the bank of Kotor Bay. And, believe it or not, there was an outdoor basketball court jutting out on a peninsula, just in front of the church. I had great fun seeing the surprised looks of the young Montenegrin men witnessing an old, white-haired, potbellied American making hook shots from halfway across the court, and blocking the shots of their local heroes. My Montenegrin hosts finally had to drag me inside to start the workshop.

People quickly dropped down into their feelings. We found the heart of conflict and violence within ourselves. There is nothing like war to inspire people to get real and reveal what is really going on within them. Most of the workshop participants were psychologists and social workers desperate to alleviate the suffering of the thousands of refugees who had escaped into their country for protection.

At one point a local psychologist expressed her sense of overwhelm at trying to meet the needs of her clients. She had several hundred refugees from the war in Bosnia in her caseload. Many of the women and children had been systematically raped by the Serbian army. As I started to empathize with her survivors' guilt, exhaustion and despair, a volcano of trapped pain erupted. She grabbed her throat as if to choke back the pain, saying, "How can I take the time to receive this empathy when others are the true victims and are suffering so much more than I?" I explained to her that just as a mother must receive nutrients in order to give milk to her young, so must healers receive the energy of empathy in order to give the healing energy of compassion to their patients.

She then allowed herself a torrent of tears as did many others in the group as they wept at the beauty of this truth. Many were released from the overwhelming sense of *responsibility for* the people suffering around them and recharged themselves with the relief that allows them to be *responsive to* the pain of others. This was a new idea for most of these helping professionals, as they too had been educated in the philosophy and psychology of self-sacrificing care for others.

Afterwards we all enjoyed a pristine sense of clarity like the sweet smell of the forest after the rain.

One young woman attending the workshop was the producer for the local radio station, Radio Kotor, and she invited me for an interview. Despite the lag of translation, the show flowed smoothly, and local interest was kindled for a new "Nonviolent Communication Community."

On the day I was scheduled to leave Montenegro, I went to the airport, only to be told that the plane would not leave till all the seats had been filled, probably the next day. My host Titsa explained that a plane reservation in Montenegro is more of a hopeful request than a firm reservation. Eventually I got back to Belgrade and began working with groups of students, teachers, psychologists and others. Each workshop was followed by a party that lasted late into the night. I have never worked or played so hard in my life.

The energy of the workshops kept building upon itself, with phenomenal peaks and valleys. At one point, two of the psychologists were giving empathy to each other about the helplessness and despair they felt about the war in their country when somehow they tapped into what seemed like the vortex of despair about the condition of the whole of humanity. Almost everyone in the room began to connect with this overwhelming hopelessness. Many broke into gut-wrenching sobs for the war, humanity and ourselves. We had tapped into what Steven Levine, the author of *Healing Into Life and Death*, calls "The Pain." At one point I physically could not hold myself up in the chair any longer. I allowed myself to fall into Nada's lap and let waves of sobs take me to the sea of endless suffering. Nada later told me that this had brought her great relief, as she was experiencing an overwhelming need to help someone, anyone. Her pain was that of the mother needing to help her suffering children. Mine was of the helpless child, devoid of hope of ever being comforted. We had dovetailing needs.

It is quite paradoxical, but within minutes of this experience, there was such an incredible connection between all of us that great hope was generated. A great sun started to shine through the frightening storm clouds. Then we had the experience of "entrainment." This is the phenomenon where a whole school of fish or birds, all headed in one direction, spontaneously turn on a dime and head in a new direction. Suddenly we all wanted to go out and party, even though it was one in the morning. And party and dance we did, in the cafes of Belgrade, until the wee hours. All of us had such a tremendous surge of energy that we had to force ourselves to finally go home and rest. All we wanted to do was joke and play and plan for new ways to bring more people into the cradle and comfort of our community of common unity. I felt the sanctity of the name the psychologists from the University of Belgrade had chosen for themselves: "The Smile Keepers."

I remember lying in my bed the next day with a smile on my face, thinking, "This would be an okay day to die, because I now know that I have really lived." I felt complete and satisfied. I could have stayed there forever, playing basketball in the morning within the walls of the castle Correymagdon, overlooking the confluence of the Sava and Danube Rivers, having profound encounters in the afternoon workshops, and celebrating intensely with my brothers and sisters into the night.

Finally the time came for me to leave, and I was sad. My mood was lightened only by the spectacle of Nada charming the train attendant first of all to let me into a packed train without a reservation, during a time of tight security. Then she managed to procure me a sleeping berth! This trick involved daring, a dash of NVC, and a heaping helping of Balkan feminine allure. Over the next weeks and months I watched the news and the progress of the revolution in Serbia. I recognized with sorrow the streets and buildings being bombed in the U.S.-led campaign to overthrow Milosevic's dictatorship. I feared I might see one of those innocent, sweet and noble Smile Keepers being carried off on a stretcher. I watched with soaring pride and hope as hundreds of thousands of Serbian demonstrators marched on Belgrade's capital demanding that Milosevic step down, withdraw the army from Kosovo, and return the government to the people. Much of the organizing for the demonstrations was done from the University of Belgrade. My Joan-of-Arc friend and sister Nada Savic was in the thick of it.

Out of the Balkan Frying Pan Into the Middle East Firestorm

The train took me back to Budapest, and from Hungary I flew to Tel Aviv, Israel, after three hours of interrogation by El Al airline security. In the process of searching my luggage, they found papers with the names of contact people in Israel—and also in the Occupied Territories. They realized that the international Center for Nonviolent Communication includes Palestinians as well as Israelis. They tore open the letters I was delivering from Smile Keepers to friends in the Middle East. They tore up most of my papers and books. I got a little preview of where U.S. security might be headed post 9-11.

Ten minutes after I got out of the interrogation room, I found myself in another very intense encounter with Israeli authorities. I turned to check out a map on the wall for a few minutes, and when I turned back a young man was clamping a lock on my bags. When I asked him what he was doing, he said, "You abandoned your bags and they are now confiscated." I said, "Wait a minute! I was just looking at that map on the wall and could not have been distracted for more than a minute or two." His body became rigid at my perceived insolence and he shouted, "So you are going to be a smart ass! You had better not interfere with police business." I was so scared that I had difficulty empathizing with him. Instead I turned into a raging jackal myself, threatening to inform his superior about his use of profanity with me. I barely got my bags back without being arrested.

Dr. Rosenberg and his "Giraffe Team" were in Israel for a week, and I joined them. We went to Betsahur in the Occupied Territories near Jerusalem and did a workshop at the Palestinian Center for Rapprochement. This organization works with young men who want to build bridges between the moderate and more radical factions. Dr. Rosenberg taught them how Nonviolent Communication could be used to create political change. This particular community was already refusing to pay their taxes, as a nonviolent protest against the presence of Israeli soldiers. The Israeli response to this was to bulldoze Palestinian houses. The Palestinians were interested in learning how to stimulate political change at lower cost to their people.

I met a young Palestinian man named Asa who invited me to spend the night with him and his family. I joined Asa and several friends on an excursion to the city's outdoor cafes, caressed by the warm winds, under the brilliant stars of the Middle Eastern sky. I felt total acceptance in the jovial company of Asa's friends and family.

Asa's father is a master woodworking artist, carving religious statues and other figures out of olive wood. However, it is difficult for him to survive financially, because Israeli law prohibits the sale of his wares. I am very proud of the hand-carved giraffe pin Asa gave me. Whenever I am feeling scared about a presentation I am going to do, like the one I did recently for sixty Episcopal ministers, I put the pin on over my heart to draw from the strength of Asa and his family. I remember their generosity in the midst of financial uncertainty. I remember their joy in community, even under military occupation. I am still deeply touched when I remember the strength of their dedication to living nonviolently in the most difficult of circumstances.

Thinking of them reminds me of why the giraffe was chosen as the symbol for Nonviolent Communication. The giraffe has the largest heart of any land animal, up to 26 lbs. It lives its life with strength, gentleness, and great vision. A part of its great vision is due to its great perspective: it sees the big picture, the whole story, from its lofty vantage point. From this larger view of the world it can see the unity of life, which inspires compassion. And because it can see the whole path, the obstacles and the destination more clearly than most, it has the confidence to continue stepping forward while others become paralyzed by self-doubt. To really live nonviolently in a violent world requires courage and compassion.

I needed that courage for the next part of my visit in the Occupied Territories. Asa took me for a ride. Driving through the streets of the ancient city was scarier than the worst roller coaster. There are no lights, lines, signs or laws. There are only a few loose traditions. Sometimes we would barrel down a street only to slam on the brakes, throw the car in reverse, and drive backwards for a half mile because the road was not wide enough to allow two cars to pass. At every corner Asa found another relative or dear friend of the family waving to him. We must have waved to two hundred people. Everyone knows everyone. There was a richness of community spirit.

From there I went back to Jerusalem where a workshop was being held to build a bridge between the Orthodox and Nonorthodox Jews, and the non-religious of Israel. It was fascinating to see how Dr. Rosenberg dealt with the absoluteness of religious belief. One Orthodox Jewish woman asked how she might get her son to follow certain rules of religious practice. Dr. Rosenberg told her to describe for her son the beauty and joy she felt following the practices and then allowing her son to take part. He told the story of the mother who brought her son to the old Rabbi because he refused to read the Torah. Instead of chastising the boy, the old Rabbi hugged him close to his heart. The boy went on to become a great Rabbinical scholar.

I was also deeply touched by the humility and delight of our host Rabbi David Zeller (the world-famous "Singing Rabbi") as he interacted with Dr. Rosenberg. Rabbi Zeller arranged a meeting between Ram Dass and Dr. Rosenberg. Ram Dass committed himself to finding more money to allow the international Center for Nonviolent Communication to train more people. Then we dined with all the old "dinosaur" Giraffes, those who have known Marshall for a long time. We had a delightful dinner with lots of laughter and teasing. At one point the wave of merriment subsided and a quieter more focused atmosphere of story telling smoothly emerged. Tales of Marshall's travels were lapped up like the most delicious dessert. All were eager for the inspiration generated by updates on the development of new Giraffe communities. Finally the news had been delivered, and it was time for questions and answers.

One of the religious Jewish giraffes asked Marshall what his Judaism meant to him. He explained the oppression and physical beatings he had suffered for being a Jew in Detroit. He told about being excluded from college fraternities because he was Jewish. Being Jewish drove him to understand the nature and causes of oppression and to seek a solution. But he looked for a solution that was not oppressive in some new way, hence Nonviolent Communication. At one point Marshall's throat filled up with emotion and his voice cracked as he said, "My Judaism means that I can never rest while anyone is oppressed." And when he said it, everyone in the room gasped and wept at the beauty of the moment. Everyone knew that for Marshall, these were not just words. He was expressing the motivation behind the last thirty-five years of this life, traveling constantly around the world teaching, with only a few days a year to rest and be with his wife and family. There is even a joke we tell whenever someone new asks us, "Where does Marshall live?" We answer, "United Airlines."

Besides the open programs for the public, there was a politics workshop. The participants were from two groups of Israeli political activists. One was a group of liberal doves, the other hawkish conservatives. Part of what made this interesting for me was that some of the people from the right wing brought guns, which they most graciously placed on a table during the workshop. It was also much less difficult than one might imagine to get each side's political analysis translated into feelings, needs and — most important — a concrete request for action.

After a couple of hours we had ferreted out several points of agreement and several agreements for action. One example:

The Right: "We are concerned about the trading of land for peace and would like you, the left, to sign a paper saying that at least the 1967 borders are non-negotiable." The left eventually agreed to this and thus found common ground with the right.

I was asked to travel north of Tel Aviv to Natanya, where a group had been practicing Nonviolent Communication for three years but had run into a block. This group lived in one of the larger kibbutzim, and were trying to create more interest in NVC, but their own internal conflicts with each other were slowing their progress. I was honored at the opportunity. The group willingly opened up and successfully moved through some very painful issues.

I was also then invited to another, nearby, smaller kibbutz of about one thousand people, to strategize about how to get NVC going there. My hostess, Ruth, was the sixty-year-old wife of a former director of the commune. I was somewhat surprised to learn that they had the same kind of communication difficulties and hurts, jealousies and guilts as small American towns. One difficulty we explored was how to deal with the hurt feelings toward people who worked outside the community, who had greater usage of the communal cars. Ruth started with a discouraged tone, "Oh yes, I got all caught up in this controversy over the automobiles. That is the last time I stick my neck out. I even wrote a letter in the community newspaper. Now some of my neighbors will not talk to me. It is very painful. I have been here thirty-five years, raised three children here, and it still seems that nobody knows how to talk about their feelings or wants without blaming, or 'guilting,' each other." They all play the game "who can get to the victim spot first." She showed me the articles in the kibbutz's newspaper where the two factions try to "out-guilt" each other. She went on to explain about the great need of the commune for Nonviolent Communication.

I taught her a technique I call, "putting up my clear plastic guilt umbrella" so the sunshine can get through but not the rain. It involves focusing my attention just on the feelings and unmet needs of the other. I suspend thinking about what I should have done differently or defending the rightness of my actions. As I was explaining this over lunch in the kibbutz's cafeteria, a young woman walked up to our cafeteria table and said to Ruth in a very hurt tone, "Oh, here you are. I thought you were supposed to be on duty in the children's library. I finally got the day care kids over to the library, and there was no one to help them because you were having a good time with this young man here." I could almost hear my hostess's heart sink with guilt. What is really sad is that this was the first time in years that my host had had a guest visit and had taken a couple of hours off duty for herself.

I empathized with my hostess's anger at hearing judgment and her guilt about taking time for herself. Ruth was then able to realize that her friend was just sending an SOS for understanding of the jealousy she was feeling that someone else was able to take some guilt-free moments of leisure. We talked about how all communication is usually either an SOS or a care package of some kind. I showed her how she might have responded to the young woman's comment instead of reacting against it. A giraffe response might have been, "Are you feeling disappointed because you really wanted the children to have some time in the library?" Ruth began to see that when we take *responsibility for* someone's pain it blocks us from being empathetically *responsive to* their pain.

It came out that this young woman had really wanted the librarian's job in the children's library and had been hurt when she was not selected. "But no one knows how to talk directly about their needs for empathy. It usually comes out like this, with someone 'justifiably' pointing the finger of shame and guilt when the opportunity arises," said Ruth with exasperation. She committed to encouraging the community leaders to invite one of the trainers from a local NVC group to do some training. She also expressed her fear that she would not be able to stay compassionate if she heard the leaders say, one more time, "We don't need this, we have God's words."

"I always lose it when I hear that sanctimonious crap, and I start thinking of them as being against change and even against me," she complained in frustration. I showed her how to give herself empathy so she could clear away the "enemy images" she carried of her community leaders. If you are seeing an authoritarian, you are being an authoritarian! Here is a song we use in some NVC workshops to illustrate how clearing away "enemy" images allows us to see each other as human:

The Gift of Empathy
by Marshall Rosenberg

I want to give you the gift of empathy

And to rid myself of lifeless thought limiting what I see.

It's taken me a while but I've come to see at last

How much I miss the present with eyes fogged by the past.

So if I take some time before I answer you.

I am clearing away my projections so your divinity can shine through.

If You Are Seeing a Jackal You Are Being a Jackal

The next day I drove up to Haifa in my rental car and had a profound encounter with a group of Israeli businessmen. Haifa is built over the top of a mountain. I was dying to play basketball so I went to the very top of the mountain where the world-famous Haifa University sits. I found my way to the gymnasium and began to play around with a couple of guys who were practicing there.

It looked as though they were about to start up a game so I turned to one of the men and asked if I could join them. He looked a little startled but then answered "Oh, no, you have to ask the big boss." And then he pointed to the biggest man on the court, standing about six feet, six inches tall, a few feet wide, and with full mustache and beard. So I went over to him, somewhat nervously, and said, with the most confidence I could muster, "The fellow over there says you are the one to ask about joining you for a game." In a thick Israeli accent the man asked, "What you want from me?" I said, "How would you feel about my playing with you for a game or two?"

"You cannot play," he said gruffly, and abruptly turned on his heel and ran to get a ball that was bouncing nearby. I felt confused for a moment as I thought to myself, "I can too play basketball, it is one of the few things I do well." I quickly realized he was denying me permission. Feeling dissatisfied with the transaction and remembering the giraffe motto, "A giraffe never gives in or gives up on his needs," I decided to persist. I walked over to where he was tying his shoe and did my best to empathize with this obviously untrue statement that I didn't know how to play basketball.

"Are you worried about getting into some kind of trouble with your boss if I play?" I asked. I was wondering if there was yet a bigger boss from which I would need to get permission. A nightmarish image flashed through my mind of an infinite line of bigger and yet bigger bosses, all with bushy beards, disappearing over the horizon. Each would deny me permission and then refer me to the next bigger boss. "It is not possible, we start the game now!" he respond-ed. And with that, he ran onto the court and started the game without me. This did not sit well with me. In fact, I was experiencing a sort of smoldering outrage, like a roaring fire with a blanket thrown over it. "How dare he?" I fumed inside, "Who the hell does he think he is? This is some way to treat a foreign guest." I sat down on the bleachers so I could watch the game as I brooded, and tried to prac-tice what Dr. Rosenberg calls "enjoying the Jackal Show" in my head, the chorus of critical thoughts. After a few minutes I began to connect with some of the needs underneath my anger: the need to be taken seriously, the need for acceptance and inclusion, the need to be valued.

-§-
If you are seeing an authoritarian you are being an authoritarian!
-§-

I thought about leaving, but shame-filled images of a whipped puppy dog with his tail between his legs prevented me. I was deter-mined to find my dignity and command, instead of demand, respect in this situation. What was this all about for me? A part of me began to connect with the hurt little boy inside that was never allowed to join his big brother and his friends when they played games. And the shame that was triggered when I internalized the interpretation, "People don't like having me around."

I wanted relief from these images so I decided to try to live by the principles of self-compassion. This would require putting myself first and only. I remembered what Steven Covey, the author of "Seven Habits of Highly Effective People," said about a lose/win (or a win/lose) really being a lose/lose. I wanted to find out what feelings and needs were behind his not wanting me to play and then "hang in" for a win/win.

After about 15 minutes the game ended and the players sat on the bleachers to rest. I walked up to the big boss, and in my best street giraffe language said, "I suspect that you are worried about getting in some kind of trouble. But I have been traveling a lot and it would be a big gift to me if you'd be willing to bend the rules and let me play." He looked up at me, astonished that I had not given up already. He said, "Look, I have orders from my boss who says no one without insurance can play." My first thought was, "Oh my God, the old insurance excuse, what a classic bureaucrat." This judgmental thought prevented me from empathizing with his message. I therefore made a too-hasty move toward a solution. I said, "But I do have insurance; in fact it is so good it covers you if you get hurt playing with me." I had also broken a cardinal rule by putting my "butt" in the face of an irritated jackal—a good way to get bitten. I later felt some amusement and some guilt about this exaggerated fabrication, but I cut myself some slack and decided it was a reflection of my desperation.

He was not amused or impressed. He simply got up and started another game with his friends. Again I felt the flare of indignation. "Where's the American Embassy? They cannot get away with this!" I mocked him in my mind, "I have orders from my boss!" As I searched my mental files for data to document the righteousness of my indignation, my mind wandered back to Jerusalem two days before. I thought of the Nazi war crimes trial in which Adolph Eichman asked, "How could you do it, give orders to gas the Jews?" He candidly explained that it was because all the officers had learned to speak "ampsprachen" (loosely translated as "bureaucratese"). Whenever questioned about why they did what they did, the standard answer was "I had to, superior's orders." In other words, blame it on your boss.

My arrogance was about to give this highly educated Jew a lesson in Jewish history when Marshall's words came back to me. He said that when you feel like lashing out, remember what the Buddha said,

"Don't just do something, sit there!" I remembered Buddha's four noble truths about what is happening when I am angry:

1. I am wanting something I am not getting.

2. I am telling myself someone should be giving it to me.

3. I am about to do something I am going to regret.

4. Even if I do shame or scare the other into giving me something, I will pay dearly for it in the long run.

Luckily, the big boss was no longer in front of me but out on the court, giving me time to give myself empathy. I began to feel the rage of my "should" thinking. My inner righteousness roared, "He should be an individual and stand up for his own values, not bow down to someone else's authority." I was completely blind to the fact that he was standing up to my authoritarianism. I began to feel all the rage and powerlessness I had felt when growing up, trying to negotiate my needs with people in authority. I felt the unresolved animosity toward my big brother, who had used his power and physical strength to dominate me. The awareness of bitter humiliation rose in my stomach as I told myself that my inability to stand up to these people meant I was a weak, cowardly, wimpy woos-woman. (How sad that my inner critic has been culturally trained to use the opposite sex as a put-down.) I felt the sadness about wanting to be included in my big brother's circle of friends. Then I felt the sadness inside me about having bought into tragic self-judgments. I grieved the loss of self-acceptance and inner strength that this shame had cost me. How sad that I had hated myself all my life for this.

Gradually a different hunger began to grow inside me. It was the hunger to see the humanity of the big boss. Up until that point I had been trying to use the technique of Nonviolent Communication with a big agenda attached. The agenda was to get him to shift his position and let me play. I had "single-mindedness of purpose," which often triggers the fear of being forced into something. Then the other becomes a mule and digs in his heels to resist, no matter what the issue. So even though I was following the letter of the principles and using the right words, "Are you feeling (worried) because you are wanting (to stay out of trouble)," the spirit of the principles of compassion was still missing. I was using the technique out of fear and confusion. The energy of real empathy was missing. I was giving "empathy from hell." But now I had empathized with and cleared away some of the hell going on inside me. I'd dropped the enemy image, and I had a genuine desire to see the human need behind the big boss's deed.

As I sat waiting for my next opportunity to "hug my demon" (which, by the way, prevents it from biting you from behind), I remembered some other things Marshall had said in the workshop in Jerusalem. He had said, "If you are seeing a jackal, you are being a jackal." I had certainly been caught up in seeing an authoritarian, bureaucratic, rigid, insensitive, buck-passing jackal-speaking jerk. And I had paid the price of slipping into the sin of judgmental thinking. I had been paying the price for years in terms of my self-created powerlessness in the face of authority figures: the psychological torment of my own rage and the simple frustration of not getting others to hear my needs. Judgmentalism is a sin with its own built-in consequence. In other words we are punished *by* this sin not *for* it.

I was feeling a different quality within myself now, one of acceptance. Previously I was thinking that the lesson was not giving in, finding a way to force my way into the game. Now I was seeing that I was already part of a much bigger game, and the lesson was to practice trusting the process. I was learning the importance of empathizing with myself trying to empathize with the other. "Get the dust out of your own eye first so you can see clearly to help get the dust out of your brother's eye," a wise Jewish man from the Middle East once said. I was becoming aware that you cannot empathize with someone because you "should," or from fear. There is an order and timing to the empathy and honesty process. If I can align myself with it, I move towards healing and wholeness.

Marshall commented on this timing issue in a workshop, when a Palestinian woman stood up and shouted, "You expect me to empathize with the Israeli soldier that shot my child?" His answer was, "Yes, but not now." She first needed to receive total empathy for the horror and grief of losing a child in that way, for the pure hate she now had for all Israelis, for the humiliation and powerlessness she felt about the political situation, and much more. Without this empathy, her other children would grow up with a mother filled with anger and hate. If she were to stay stuck in the thinking of racial hatred for all Israelis, she would be contributing to the political climate that led to the death of her child in the first place. (I also believe that cancers, ulcers and other medical complications are created or reinforced by unresolved emotional pain.)

By the time the big boss came back to rest on the bleachers, I was excited about making my own contribution to world peace by healing the conflict within me about powerful authority figures. I suspect he was expecting me by this time. "I am a little nervous saying this," I began, "but I do understand that you are concerned about doing what your boss wants you to. However, I am worried that if I leave without coming to a better resolution, I will regret it. I would like you to reconsider allowing me to play."

"Look, I have children to feed and I am not going to risk losing my job," said the burly man, this time making direct eye contact with me. It was then that the most amazing metamorphosis occurred, lifting me above the maze of separateness and into the clarity of our common humanity. Suddenly I felt a surge of compassion and clarity of connection to the huge heart of a fellow giraffe just trying to protect his children's food supply. Where I had seen rigidity, I now saw fierce love for his children. Where I had seen authoritativeness, I now saw passionate self-confidence. What I had judged as insensitivity was now a beatific self-compassion. I felt a wave of great admiration and caring for the man for taking such precious care of his children.

I also felt the shift of resolution inside me that had nothing to do with compromise. Now I was one hundred percent clear that I no longer wanted to play basketball if it meant that this loving father would have anxiety about the well-being of his children.

They started another game and again I sat on the bleachers to process my feelings. Overwhelming feelings of gratitude and joy gushed up from deep within me in, while waves of tears flowed down my face. I remembered a song title a friend wrote: "I saw world peace flowing down your cheek." I proved within myself that if you keep dancing with a jackal long enough, it really does start to grow giraffe spots. Marshall was right when he said, "There really aren't any jackals—just giraffes with a language challenge." I was grateful to myself that I had trusted the process long enough to see through my judgmental projections to get to that other world of a compassionate understanding of the unity of all life. All I wanted to do was to sit and feel the waves of hope and relief.

Then the voice of the big boss boomed across the court, "I go now. I no longer want to play." He had come up with a synergistic "Shultz solution." Remember Sergeant Shultz from the TV show "Hogan's Heroes"? Whenever Colonel Hogan was doing something against the rules, that Shultz was supposed to stop, he would put a hand over his eyes and declare, "I see nothing, absolutely nothing."

I looked up as he walked out of the gym. The other nine men, who had been sympathetic all along to my wanting to play, now looked over at me with smiles in their eyes. They did not have to say a word. I jumped up and ran onto the court. "Which team am I on?" I asked. Inside I knew, at least in that moment, that we are all on the same team.

One enemy image got transformed that day into an affirmation of our brotherhood in our common humanity. But why is it so difficult to do? Where do all these enemy images come from? What are they costing us individually, spiritually and as a nation in the world? These enemy images play out as conflicts in our love relationships, in our communities and on the world stage. The same forces are at work my local individual encounter in the Middle East, and in America's global interactions in the post-9/11 world.

A Few Bad Apples? Or a Barrel of Rotting Culture?

U.S. General Taguba found that between October and December of 2003 there were numerous instances of "sadistic, blatant, and wanton criminal abuses" at Abu Ghraib prison in Iraq by American forces. The American Red Cross says that these abuses were wide spread in prisons all over Iraq and Afghanistan and that they tried, unsuccessfully for many months to get our government to stop it.

How could we, the United States of America, land of the free and home of the brave produce young men and women who rape, sodomize, torture and beat to death God only knows how many innocent Iraqi men, women and teenagers? Is it really just a "few bad apples" as our military and government explain? Or could it be the vinegar barrel of our still evolving culture and institutions that is producing people who are all too willing, in fact are photographed smiling, as they torture and humiliate other human beings?

I am not interested in blaming the current administration or getting more people punished higher up the chain of command. Punishment is the problem not the solution. It is precisely the belief that "us" good guys are being noble by punishing "them" bad guys that allowed our soldiers to commit such acts in the first place. It is our U.S. belief in retributive justice (see "Revenge"), and making sure that people get what they deserve, that is the philosophical foundation for wanting to make people suffer.

One commanding officer was asked whether he tried to influence the politics of the soldiers under his command to support or not support the war. He said "Never. I just tell them to remember what Bin Laden did to us." No agenda there.

I am coining a new word "Enemyism" which, like its cousin racism, creates a perspective, a set of glasses to look thru, that transforms a human being into an object, an enemy to be hated, feared and punished. When we are carry such enemy images we cannot then at the same time be wholly aware of our own needs, say for security.

Enemyism creates a sense of superiority and therefore separateness. This superiority makes the other less valuable and therefore expendable. (When Pentagon officials were asked how many civilian men, women and children were killed the answer was "We do not keep track of collateral damage.") Notice the use of semantics to obscure the truth. Enemyism not only demonizes the bad "other" it sanitizes the good "us" (see "U.S."). They are "terrorists" we are "liberators".

Another part of Enemyism is our cultural myth that being "good" means being a destroyer of evil. This can really disguise our own vengeful motives from ourselves. Then when the right stressful situation occurs. Boom! It explodes out of the repressed dark side of our psyche. This prison abuse scandal is an explosion out of the repressed dark side of our cultural psyche. This dark side justifies revenge and hurting people by saying it is done for "good."

In order to maintain a Warrior/Dominator culture you have to make violence good, honorable, heroic, and noble. I remember working with young Palestinian men at the Center for Rapprochement in Betsahur, in the Occupied Territories of the Middle East. (Palestine). When we got to understand the needs that made suicide bombings look like a good idea, it sounded like something straight out of West Point. They explained that they would do it out of love of their country, for honor and to show their mothers and sisters that they loved them. So maybe the grand difference between us and them is not so grand, but I believe it could be. If we could use this great, great opportunity to look at ourselves and to decide that if we don't like what we see in the mirror to change it. Like that other guy from the middle east who said something like "You have been taught eye for an eye and a tooth for a tooth. I bring you a new covenant." We need a new covenant as ours is clearly not working.

Top 10 reasons I am not surprised to hear that our sweet young U.S. men and women sexually tortured and killed, captive, helpless Iraqis:

1. Their central cultural myth supported such actions. In all our history books the good American hero kills its bad enemies. The good

guys hurt the bad guys for good reasons. And our media desensitizing us to violence, making it heroic and enjoyable as the hero kills or beats up someone in 75% of prime time TV shows. This happens at the "climax" of the movie and is rewarded with winning the girl. This is all part of the eroticization of violence and it is therefore not at all surprising that so much of the prisoner abuse was linked with sexuality. (If you doubt our U.S. enjoyment of the macabre, go to a Texas tailgate party. You can find one any time someone is about to be executed in Texas. There is much drinking and celebration in anticipation of what Dr. Rosenberg calls 'the magic moment'. The moment when they announce that the prisoner is dead, which is followed by many raucous Yahoo's and Yipee's.)

2.   Their central cultural paradigm supported their actions. Bad people (i.e. those Iraqis arrested by the army) deserve to suffer and be punished by us good people. It is OK to use power over tactics if it is for a "good" (translate: One I think I am right about.) cause. Power over tactics include coercion, punishment, reward, threats, guilt, shame, and duty. The side effect of the constant use of power over tactics to "shape" good behavior in U.S. institutions is a self absorbed citizen, who primarily thinks about whether a certain action will get punished or a rewarded. This thinking prevents empathy, compassion or awareness of how our actions actually affect others. It is a self centered morality. From this perspective following orders to abuse people is the smart thing to do.

3.   Their compulsory education (an oxymoron in itself) process supported the needed psychology to do what they did. It taught them to think in terms of moralistic judgments, i.e. in terms of what people "are". This thinking reduces human beings, oneself and others, to objects and into categories like slow and gifted, A students and C students, moral and immoral, patriotic and unpatriotic, mentally ill and normal, good and bad, right and wrong. School testing then reinforces that you deserve to be where you are and you get what you deserve. This maintains a Domination caste system disguised to look like a democracy. It is likely our soldiers were unconsciously expressing the rage and humiliation of this dehumanizing process, then justifying it

by thinking that they just gave those "terrorist" prisoners "what they deserved."

4. They were trained to "think like machines" under stressful authoritarian competitive conditions in order to beat their fellow student opponents on their SATs. (Standardized Testing = Standardized Thinking). In Michael Lerner's book *Spirit Matters* he says "Nothing eliminates a sense of connection to others more effectively than the way contemporary schooling teaches students that their own success depends on their ability to do better than others." This loss of a sense of connection to others drains emotional strength and destroys one's ethical compass. And besides thinking for oneself and having empathy for others is easily seen as a threat to the "chain of command". If they had been trained to think for themselves and stay connected to their hearts and empathy for others, the mob mentality could not have gotten rolling.

5. Their public school and cultural training supported the dulling of awareness of their own freedom of choice. Our Dominator culture punishes us if we don't do what authority says is right, and uses language that hides the truth that we have a choice. This language sounds like *should, have to, must, can't, had to* and is the very language Adolph Eichmann says made it easy for him to kill millions of Jews. (According to the book Eichmann in Jerusalem, by Arendt, at his war crimes trial he called this language Amtssprache, in German. He said everyone used this responsibility denying language, saying "I had no choice, superior's orders." How interesting that this is the exact same defense and words the lawyers for the soldiers accused in the Abu Ghraib incident, are now using.) Our soldiers were never taught the difference between respect for authority and obedience to authority.

6. I took psychology 101. Here I learned that Stanley Milgram of Yale University found that 65% of "normal." Americans will deliver apparently lethal electric shocks of 450 volts-to a pitifully screaming, protesting innocent victim, simply because an authority commanded them to. The research also found that if one of the researchers labeled the subjects (by calling them "animals") they greatly increased the

willingness to use more voltage more often. When our supposedly objective media, our compassionate conservative President, our government, our military leaders and practically our whole culture uses dehumanizing labels like terrorists, insurgents, militants, enemy fighters, criminals, evil doers, etc., what do we think is going to happen?

7. The soldiers were given a good "cover story." The Milgram study researchers found that if they gave a good "cover story" like "you are not hurting helpless people, you are helping eager learners learn by shocking them" this too increased the willingness to use of more voltage more often. You are not imprisoning and killing tens of thousands of innocent men, women and children, (The Red Cross says 90% of those in prisons are there by mistake) you are liberating people from oppression so it does not matter how you do it. Of course you have to believe in the concept "the ends justifies the means." One way this is taught to U.S. children is through physically beating them while suggesting "this is for your own good." The prison guard soldiers were given the "cover story" that torturing their captives would help get information that could save U.S. lives. Our government tells us we need to go to war and give up freedoms for the sake of "national security".

8. I took psychology 102. Here I learned about Dr. Philip Zimbardo's extensive research showing that average Americans (screened for criminal behaviors, or mental problems) when asked to role play guards of a made up prison, if not checked, will become sadistic torturers after a few days. In fact the experiments had to be stopped because of the increasing violence and sexual content of the guards actions. "When people are deindividualized, they are usually put in herds, or groups, and given numbers, their identity is taken away," Zimbardo said. "[In Abu Ghraib] the guards had a mob mentality, a group mindset. The results are predictable." You can tell what people have been made of, their deep cultural programming, when you put them in a stressful situation. (Both Milgram and Zimbardo's work has resurfaced in mainstream media programs like ABC News Nightline.) People growing up in a culture of empathy and respect for autonomy could not do what our young men and women did.

9. They were misrecognized. Our institutions teach people develop "useful" validatable skills in order to "earn" recognition, caring and support. They teach people to ignore pleasure, nurturance, our interconnectedness and the awesome wonder of our inner spiritual nature. Author Michael Lerner says the children labeled "dysfunctional" have not learned to hide the pain and anger of not being seen for themselves. The "successful" children develop a split between their inner and outer selves. These successful children become our soldiers, but with a deep hole in their soul and hunger for recognition. This hunger manifested as a willingness to do unspeakable things in order to "belong" to the group and to "earn" the approval of their commanders.

10. They had no way of thinking or speaking about the prisoners in a humane way. Why do the soldiers and our politicians keep using these polarizing, inflammatory judgments? Of course there are many reasons, some political, religious and due to their domination culture socialization. However I also believe it is because of the ignorance of the connection between this dehumanizing labeling and acts of violence. Our culture basically has no way of thinking or speaking about people who are operating outside our value system or not meeting our needs without demonizing them. This is why I think the principles for speaking and thinking that the Nonviolent Communication teachings make clear are the most desperately needed commodity on the planet to create realistic security.

Chapter

BECOMING A NON-RUSHIN' UNORTHODOX

If you don't have time to read this, you should convert to my new religion: Non-Rushin' Unorthodox. An important part of evolving my selfishness is developing a more hedonistic relationship with time. I have not been getting all my needs met in my relationship with time, and I now choose to be more assertive about them. The primary need I have is to enjoy my time.

And so I am going to take my time as I write this chapter. Why? Because I have been a-rushin' most all my life and I'm bone tired. Rushin' to get through school, rushin' to build a private practice, rushin' to find someone to love. All so that I could stop rushing and relax. What I am discovering is that my mind always finds something more to rush about. Now my mind wants me to hurry up and write this book. My mind says, "Then I'll let you have some peace."

Well, I have finally named that mental voice for the sneaky serpent it is. Yes, I have finally seen the light, praise God, and I've become a born again Non-Rushin' Unorthodox. (Or maybe I should call it "The Church of the Later-in-the-Day Saints.") In my religion there is only one sin: To rush. It is moral to move at great speeds, but not to rush. In fact the faster you are moving the more dangerous it is to rush. Just ask one of our more prominent church members Dale Earnhardt of NASCAR fame. But there is a big difference between rushing and moving at the speed needed to achieve your goal.

A couple of weeks ago I was driving to a workshop I was to give in Los Angeles. I had started out forty-five minutes after I would have liked because I was rushing around trying to get a lot of things done before I left. The workshop was to start at three p.m., and at my present rate of speed, sixty five mph, I figured I would be arriving at 3:45 p.m.

Notice I did not say I would be forty-five minutes late. That's because "late" is a four letter word for a Non-Rushin' Unorthodox. In Non-Rushin' Seminary Schools it is a debate of phenomenological proportions as to whether "late" even has existential existence. Sure, some people arrive at meetings after other people want them to. But we have to have cultural collusion between at least two people to agree that someone is late. "Late" has no independent existence. Therefore a Non-Rushin' Unorthodox is never late. Late is a cultural abstraction. In some cultures the concept of late does not exist, and there are great differences about what late means in other cultures. For example, when I held workshops for psychologists at the University of Belgrade, in Serbia, the workshop would be scheduled to start at six p.m., and no one would even start showing up until nine p.m. I am glad I didn't think of them as being late or else I would have been furious.

Because I had not yet been truly saved from the evils of rushing, I was completely wrapped up in the coils of that serpent called "Anxiety" as I sped toward Los Angeles. As I imagined the people at the workshop angrily tapping their feet and looking at their watches, I felt a sickening surge of adrenaline rise in my stomach. My foot would lunge forward on the gas. Then I would look up into the rear view mirror and hallucinate someone's roof top luggage rack into a police car's blue flashing light and quickly back off the accelerator. I was caught between the braking effect of the fear of getting yet another speeding ticket, and the accelerating effect of the anxiety of being late.

Just then an enchanting song came on the radio and for a moment I lost track of the two pendulums of peril I was caught between. As soon as the song ended, I noticed the pull of my imagination: out the window of my car, down I-5 and into the room of angry, impatient seminar participants. The familiar feeling of anxious doom raised its ugly head as I visualized them walking out of the room in disgust. As soon as I returned my mind's eye to the trees on the side of the road, the shiny red truck in the next lane, and to my present thoughts about how interesting this all was, I could feel the swell of anxiety recede. I realized that, "Wow, if I could just keep my thoughts and visualizing inside the car, I would feel a lot better." Moving through space in a car is like traveling through time. To the degree I could keep my attention on things I presently controlled, things that were inside the car, the radio, air conditioning, my thoughts, I felt peaceful. As my mind tried to cross bridges it had not yet come to and do its suffering ahead of time, I felt miserable. Could old Ram Dass have been right with all that "Be Here Now" stuff?

Because I had been so focused on "being here now" for most of the drive, when I did arrive forty-five minutes after the time my seminar was scheduled, I arrived with presence — meaning that I arrived without fear, guilt, or thoughts of the past or future. I arrived with confidence and awareness of what was called for in the moment.

I needed it. As I walked into the classroom to do my seminar, three-fourths of the participants groaned with disappointment. It was a group of Latino high school students. They were not happy about being forced to attend a seminar on Nonviolent Communication. They also seemed upset about the time I was arriving. So I asked "How many of you are annoyed about the time I am arriving?" Three honest souls raise their hands. I pointed to the toughest-looking young man and asked, "What is it about my coming at three forty-five instead of three that annoys you?"

"Well, it's like this," he says as he pulls his hands out from under his arms and starts to make exaggerated gang gestures, "Adults think that kids' time doesn't matter. It's like all that's important is adults' time and to heck with the kids."

"So you are annoyed because you would have liked your time respected?" I asked.

"Yeah, man."

"And what about you?" I pointed to the one girl who had raised her hand.

"Like nobody even bothered to tell us, like it don't matter," she protested in her thick Latina accent.

"Yeah, you would have at least liked to have been told what the hold-up was?" I empathized.

And so the dialogue went for about twenty minutes, much to the fascination of the rest of the students in the classroom. After I had empathized with the students to their satisfaction, I asked them if they would like to hear what had caused me to arrive at three forty-five. Some seemed interested. I briefly explained about all the anxiety and overwhelm and fear that was going on in my life. I told them how I had got caught up rushing around, and left San Diego much later than I wanted to.

-§-
If I change my image of you, you cannot help but change your image of me. Also I will feel less scared of you as soon as I image the human feelings and needs behind your actions.
-§-

One young man was able to empathize in his own way, "Yeah, I am like that in finals week where I am so scared about getting all this studying done that I am late to the test, which really messes me up."

This was the beginning of my conversion to being a *fun*-damentalist true believer in Non-Rushin' Unorthodoxy. I saw the uselessness and pain of projecting myself into the future.

At this point, you may be wondering, "But what about planning and preparing for the future?" I want to make a distinction between anxiety-provoking catastrophic thinking related to rushing, and other, more productive kinds of thinking. These might be called preparing, planning, or analyzing a problem.

For example, I factored in the flow of traffic, weighed the risk of getting a speeding ticket, and estimated how much earlier I would get there if I drove seventy instead of sixty-five. Then I performed what felt like a powerful act of self-care. I moved my cruise control from sixty-five to seventy.

You might ask, "Now wait a minute! Aren't you starting to rush now?" I would reply, "No I am not. Rushing is a state of consciousness, not a particular external action." I can walk at my top speed and not be rushing. Or I can walk at half my top speed and be totally caught up in the raging ravages of the river of rushing.

The great learning theorist, Piaget, says that all learning is a series of key differentiations. Refining our discrimination allows us more choices, and more effective choices. Planning for and doing acts of preparation must be differentiated from beating the worry drums, worry, worry...worry, worry... about the future, hoping to keep the evil spirits of misfortune away. Worrying is an abandonment of oneself. When I worry I lose awareness of my present needs and possible nurturing actions I could take for myself. I leave myself behind as my imagination takes me into an unreal, unnecessary and unhealthy future. Converting anxiety into actions to address the future is being a good parent to oneself. Here's a traveling tip from Triple A: "One Antidote for Anxiety is Action."

The power of taking action is that it begins to return you to the present by giving you feedback from your environment which can help you relocate your center. Taking action moves you back toward that state sometimes called "flow." Eckhart Tolle confirms this idea in his book *The Power of Now* when he says,

> Any action is often better than no action, especially if you have been stuck in an unhappy situation for a long time. If it is a mistake, at least you learn something, in which case it is no longer a mistake. If you remain stuck, you learn nothing. Is fear preventing you from taking action? Acknowledge the fear, watch it, take your attention into it, be fully present with it. Doing so cuts the link between the fear and your thinking.

Don't let the fear rise up into your mind. Use the power of the Now. Fear cannot prevail against it.

You First. Time Can Wait

Stephen Covey, in his book *First Things First,* talks about being addicted to anxiety and urgency. He says there are true emergencies like when a fireman goes to a fire. One reason people become firemen is for the excitement and the sense of importance and purpose they experience on a daily basis. Then there are artificial emergencies: getting caught up in the everyday rat race, fueled by fears of not having enough, of not surviving. Perhaps our longing for this sense of purpose and importance keeps us creating urgencies. After all, if you are rushing around doing urgent things, don't you look and feel more important?

-§-
If I give empathy to make another feel better, it is rarely empathy. It is often anxiety.
-§-

If I have a cell phone, pager, voice mail, web site, palm top, laptop and e-mail, that means my time is sought after and therefore I am valuable. Maybe if I rush around fast enough I can stay ahead of the Edgar Allen Poe ghost voice that says, "You're wasting your time, you're not getting ahead, you are going to die with great weeping and wailing and gnashing of teeth because you blew it!" What a nightmare! No, No, No, stop it all! Wake up!

See the light and become a Non-Rushin' Unorthodox. Convert yourself from a fear-based attitude of hustling for food, to a self-caring attitude based on tending the garden of your life. (F.E.A.R. = fantasized experiences appearing real). Here's a poem that reminds me to do this:

Take Time
by Patty Zeitlin

Maybe there's really no such thing as time, baby.
Maybe there's really no such thing as time, maybe.
Tickety-tock, we've invented the clock, we've got time, or do we?
Tickety-tock, we've invented the clock, we've got time.

Take time to smell the flowers,
Take time to look at the stars,
Take time to feel the rain on your face,
Give up the race and take time.
Take time to write a letter,
Take time to visit a friend.
Take time to learn a song that you like.
Take time. It's yours to spend.
Take time to walk and wander.
Take time for life's mysteries.
Take time to follow through on your dreams,
No matter how crazy it seems, take time.
Take time, if you remember,
Take time in every day,
Take time to care for all that you love.
There's plenty of time,
But it slips away.

One way to start taking time is to put your serenity first and refuse to rush. As I said before, this does not preclude your moving as fast as you need to in order to get to places at the time you want to. It does require you to focus on being gentle with yourself, trusting that there is enough time and giving time to what is really important, like prioritizing, planning, preparing, protection and care of the soul.

Fear-less Living

"But what about when you really do need to hurry, like when you are late for an appointment?" you ask. Believe it or not, you still have real choices available to you. You could, for example, follow my example. Recently I was running late for an appointment with an editor and started to panic. You know that feeling when you look at the clock and realize that even if you are able to break the land speed record, you will still be at least ten minutes late—and that is if the parachute on your car opens so you don't overshoot your target. I sometimes have that paralyzed octopus amputee feeling, where I have eight things I need to do first, and in perfectly prioritized order, but I only have two arms left.

Driving to meet the editor, my brain cells were busy processing catastrophic contingencies. What if the editor gets insulted and fires me? Or worse, what if she keeps me but decides to take it out on me over the next ten years by sabotaging my writing? In this state of near brain-death, I drove right past my freeway exit.

I am sure you have your own similar story to tell. Everybody agrees that haste makes waste. But then why is rushing still so popular? I think it is because it appears to pay. It looks like you really do get to work a few minutes earlier than you would have, and that your boss is three percent less angry with you than she would otherwise have been.

But what if you could get the same payoff at lower cost? What if you could walk into your workplace with an aura of peace and presence that would inspire connection instead of criticism? Because unexpressed fear often appears to other people as an expression of guilt or aggression, it can elicit criticism. So when you walk into your office filled with anxiety caused by rushing around, you are not only more vulnerable to criticism, you are more likely to get it. It is similar to the attack dog that smells fear in someone and is inspired to bite them.

The Hurrieder You Go, the Behinder You Get

Oprah asked author M. Scott Peck, "How do you find the time to do all that you do? You are a best-selling author of several books, the director of the Foundation for Community Encouragement, as well as a lecturer, therapist, and husband. How do you do it?" Scott Peck replied, "I spend a lot of time each day doing nothing." And Archbishop Desmund Tutu once said "I have so much I want to do today I better spend another hour in prayer." How appropriate that he was awarded the Nobel Peace Prize.

When I'm rushing I have outrun my soul, like a cartoon in which the character takes off, running so fast he leave his shoes (soles and all) behind. So one of the first important steps to becoming a Non-Rushin'

Unorthodox is to repent and feel the sorrow of your sins. How sad that you and I have lived in so much fear all our lives. Always running, like the scared rabbit in Alice in Wonderland: "I'm late, I'm late, for a very important date!" How sad that we have not noticed the cost that our addiction to urgency has had on our lives. What a cost to our creativity, productivity and efficiency! How sad that I did not take the time to take in what my Pennsylvania Dutch uncle told me many years ago, "The hurrieder you go, the behinder you get."

Once we are in touch with the painful cost of rushing, and are really grieving, then we are ready to receive the First (and only) Commandment in the Non-Rushin' Unorthodox Religion.

Thou shalt not rush.

The Cardinals and I are thinking about adding another Commandment to the list. By "Cardinals" I don't mean the bigwigs at the Vatican, who are ordained into red suits. I mean the *real* cardinals that already have red suits on, plus wings and feathers. I meet and meditate with these cardinals every morning for breakfast. They eat the birdseed that I put out, and I eat toast, drink coffee, and write. Here's the second commandment we're considering:

Thou shalt not be busy.

It is okay to have a full schedule of pleasurable and satisfying activities, but it is not okay to cross the line into the sacrilege of busy-ness.

Be careful not to skip over the repenting part because

> It takes a lot of grieving
> To be open to receiving.

Receiving what? The kingly luxury of realizing that there is never a need to rush. You never saw Yul Brenner rush, in his role as the King of Siam. No, he took big slow steps across the stage as he pondered life and love's deepest complexities etc, etc, etc. The world waited on him!

Celebracy

It takes commitment and consciousness to maintain my vow of Celebracy. All us priests in the Non-Rushin' Unorthodox religion take a vow of Celebracy. We stay in celebration of the present moment—NOW! I broke my vow recently while waiting in line at the movie theater. It was a very long line and they had one ticket window open with one blond, eighteen year old girl working it. The temptation was great and, I felt justified. In my moment of weakness I began to indulge in the fornication of agitation: "Why don't they open another window? It's because they know we are over a barrel and they are too greedy and cheap to pay another five-dollar-an-hour employee."

I can really work myself up in these situations. When I notice I am losing control, I can regain control by surrendering to the loss of control. It is like when your car goes into a skid on an icy road. They tell you to turn toward the slide. Since I am indulging in righteousness anyway, I sometimes take control by adding fuel to the fire of my aggravation with thoughts of annihilation: "So you corporate communists at Mann Theaters think you're The Man. I'll show you who's The Man!" So now my mind is really out of control. What am I feeling? Furious! What's under that? Powerlessness and fear. What are the needs related to the powerlessness and fear? I want to be able to have some control in the situation to be able to affect it. I want to take care of my needs. What are my needs? To value my time.

-§-
Are you hearing the truth of the moment, or having a flashback from the past? Notice it and acknowledge it.
-§-

Now that I have my mind focused in needs language, instead of justifiable murderous mental masturbation, I can begin to problem-solve by looking for ways to meet my present needs, and/or learn from the situation to care for myself better in the future. This also meets my present need to make valuable use of my time right now by engaging in problem-solving: "Maybe I could take advantage of this opportunity to network." (My friend Ann Boe, author of *Is Your Net Working,* got on the Donahue show by networking in the few seconds she waited for an elevator door to open.) Or, "Next time I go to a movie or the DMV, or the doctor's office, or anywhere I might have to wait, I am going to bring either a book or a writing tablet." It is really a joy these days to be able to keep my vow of Celebracy, and live in the non-altered state of the devout non-rushin,' by bringing a book along to read or a notebook to write in. While everyone else at line in the bank is consumed with sweating the small stuff, I am celebrating that I am not. Instead I am basking in a consciousness of Rest, a state of peace that passeth all understanding.

I like the way Rev. Deborah L. Johnson, author of *Letters from the Infinite* and president of the Inner Light Ministries, writes about this special place of peace and Rest that always exists even in the eye of the hurricane. She writes "You can get Rest from me [meaning God] even in the midst of a seemingly hectic or busy schedule. This Rest is a state of being. What do I mean when I say that it is a state of being? A state of being refers to a condition of consciousness. A state of being reflects a consciousness that is continuous. It is not in the particular; instead, it infuses every thought, word, and deed. You can take it with you wherever you go."

Putting It Into Practice

Every distressing thought or situation is an opportunity to perfect my selfishness and figure out how to either get what I want or want what I am getting. I cannot do this if I am not accepting what is happening, or if I am up in my head judging, analyzing or fearfully fantasizing. And I am clearly "in denial" any time I am thinking "should" as in "this should not be happening" or "that should be happening." I am denying "What Is," and instead I need to notice what I am feeling. Noticing feelings will help me get conscious of what I am needing, so I can decide whether to Accept the situation, Assert my needs, or Abandon the situation. (Again notice the clever triple A.)

When I'm rushing, it's like I'm in a bad dream. Somehow I'm behind in some race for my life and I can never quite seem to catch up, yet the race goes on and on. Sometimes the dream is filled with paranoia that something is chasing me. What? The fear of wasting my precious time, or is it simply death? I'm really afraid of being caught up in fear. The fear that makes me rush comes from a fantasy image I'm holding in my mind. Stan Dale, the founder of The Human Awareness Institute, describes it this way: "Fear is the dark room in which you develop your negatives."

When I rush, I'm holding images like, "Not having enough time," or "Running out of time," or "Missing an important opportunity," or creating some catastrophic consequence for myself. When I rush I am always projecting some painful outcome into the future.

A new technique I've been using lately is this: when I catch myself having that rushing feeling, I speed up. Yes, I speed up. I've found it takes more concentration to do things faster, which makes it more difficult to think about other things, like future fear fantasies. For example, I am washing dishes and if I notice I am rushing I will decide to really concentrate on being really careful not to break any, but also become more efficient with each movement. Gradually I increase the speed and see how focused and efficient I can be without clanging pans or breaking dishes. This helps to bring me back into the present where no rushing rushnecks live.

To be a Non-Rushin' devotee, design your own unique wake-up call, and use it each time you catch yourself rushing. When I am puttering around the house and notice a queasy anxiety in my shoulders, which lets me know I am starting to rush, I sing myself the first two bars from this song:

Life's Sweet Flow
by Marshall Rosenberg

I like being aware that there's nothing to achieve.
Life's a gift I have only to receive.
And I want to stay in touch with life's sweet flow,
And spread loving waves wherever I go.
I want everything I say or do,
To bring strength, warmth, and light to you.

All life must become puttering. Just say "No" to self-inflicted deadlines, or expectations about how much you're supposed to get done. Say "No" to illusions of the scarcity of time. When you're caught up in the expectation that you need to be doing more, then commit to getting less done. Take the time to find you again. "Now, let's see: Where did I put me? There I am, in the closet behind all my fears." My fears say, "If you don't live up to these imaginary expectations, I'm going to beat you up bad." So come on out of there and be here now. As Los Vegas casinos declare, "You must be present to win!"

You Might Be a Rushneck

Take a look at the list below and think about your typical behaviors. You might be a Rushneck if:

- You multi-multi-task. You talk on your cell phone while eating a fast food taco, listening to a tape on stress reduction, pressing your thigh master, drying your nails out the car window, and thinking about whether you should buy that timeshare in Utah.

- You were subpoenaed to testify as part of the Tailgate investigation.

- You skimmed any part of this chapter.

- Yesterday you were caught in rush hour traffic so you didn't stop for gas. Today you're going to be late for work if you stop for gas, and desperately late if you run out of gas.

- You're in a hurry to get to a lecture entitled "Finding Inner Peace."

- You're caught in a game of Rushin' Roulette.

- You are leaning forward when you are driving as if to get your nose across the finish line first, in case of a photo finish.

- You are willing to engage in only threeplay, or twoplay, before sex.

- You take more than thirteen shortcuts to work.

Take the Time
by Kelly Bryson

Take the time. Take the time.
You're neither fast nor slow.
Take the time. Take the time.
Because it's yours you know.

What's the worry? What's the hurry?
You're missing the moment now.
Just slow down. Look around.
Trust shows the way and how.

Don't pedal faster, 'cause what you're after
It's in the scenery, that's all around.
Just slow down, look around. It's waiting to take you in.
I want to change my goal from getting there
To enjoying myself everywhere.
Along the way, learn to stay
Fully engaged in each day.
It's a cosmic joke this thing called ambition.
To enjoy myself is my new mission.
I want to know what the sparrow knows.
Doesn't worry 'bout food or clothes.
He just accepts what he is given.
Doesn't worry 'bout making a livin'.
Just keeps singing out his sweet song.
'Bout livin' fully all day long.

Take the time. Take the time.
You're neither fast nor slow.
Take the time. Take the time.
Because it's yours you know.

Chapter

BEWARE OF THE NICE THERAPIST

Since depression is frequently a result of excessive niceness, many nice people often find themselves seeking out therapists to talk to. Most therapists, unfortunately, have been trained to be very nice themselves. The problem with nice therapists is that as soon as you're not making the progress they think you should be, Dr. Jekyll becomes Mr. Hyde.

Remember Dr. Hannibal "the cannibal" Lechter, the truly "psycho" therapist in the movie classic "The Silence of the Lambs"? Jodie Foster interviews him in prison and asks him why he had killed and eaten several of his psychotherapy clients. To which he responded, "I did them a favor; they were going nowhere in their therapy." From the safety of the other side of prison bars, the Oscar-winning Foster challenges him, "Turn your highly developed power of perception toward yourself, doctor, if you're not too scared of what you will find."

Anna Freud once said, "I love being a therapist. It is by far the best psychological defense mechanism I've found." As a state licensed therapist myself, if someone tells me I am full of myself, I simply point out the obvious insecurity they feel around people with high self-esteem.

If they then say to me 'Aren't you being a little judgmental there?' I laugh at them heartily and point out how blind they are to the enormity of their hypocrisy—not to notice that calling me judgmental is a judgment.

Unfortunately for us therapists and our loved ones, our defense system is the socially and medically accepted standard for diagnosing others. This makes it very difficult for us to notice when we are stuck in our stuff, projecting blame and denying our own responsibility, very nicely, of course. The American Medical Association, the American Psychiatric Association and several others all agree that not only does our stuff not stink, it is also scientifically correct. We have no way to let go of our stuff, and so we become spiritually and psychologically constipated. I have worked with quite a few spouses of therapists who have been driven to distraction through maddening dialog with their partners. Can you imagine having a partner who has been trained to see other people's behavior in terms of what is sick? These professionals have been taught not to reveal their own reactions, but to stay cool, calm, logical and analytical of others. I wonder what the murder rate is in couples where one is a therapist?

Some therapist friends of mine love to complain to me how most of their clients are stuck in a cycle of constantly complaining, a "complaint constipation." When their clients do it, they call it "playing victim." When they are complaining to me about their clients, they call it "healthy venting." They talk about how helpless, frustrated and irritated they are when their clients refuse to assume their own power. Hmm… "Do you ever feel victimized by your client's victim-hood?" I ask. This rarely goes over well, but some dissociated angry part of myself enjoys their discomfort with my inquisition.

I suspect my therapist friends feel helpless when their clients are expressing their helplessness and fear of change. And because they are dissociated (of course they would call this a healthy, objective, professional or Zen detachment) from their own feelings of helplessness, they become irritated whenever their clients start "playing victim." It's okay to tell your client to "vent" their feelings, even negative ones, but it is therapeutically taboo to "dump" any of your feelings on the client. This is part of the therapist's prohibition against expressing any feelings, for fear of being diagnosed as engaging in transference. As a therapist, you are only allowed to model the needless, wantless, patient, people-pleasing perfect parent. (I am reminded of a line from a song I sing which says "To give is domination if I can't also receive.") The client then tries and tries to emulate this saint-like, all-giving, never-receiving therapist, only to fail to measure up again and again. I have clients who have tried to talk to their therapists about this dynamic, and run into the classic double blind block.

They ask their therapist something like, "I'm a little confused and worried about something. I show you a lot of my vulnerability and feelings, but I don't remember you ever showing me any of yours. Are you concerned at all about the level of honesty in our relationship?" Depending on the school the therapist went to here is what might come back:

The Humanistic Nondirective: "So you're confused and worried that you show me your vulnerability and feelings, but you don't remember me showing any of mine," is the maddening, parrot-phrasing echo from the actively listening therapist. He sits there with such a warm, understanding face, fatherly angora button-up sweater, and empathetic eyes, that you'd feel guilty if you smacked him.

Author Sidney Jourard was one of my first professors of psychology at the University of Florida. In his book *The Transparent Self* he expressed his feelings about being trained as a nondirective therapist this way:

> I was quite well-trained in two main schools of psychotherapeutic theory and technique: the client-centered approach of Carl Rogers and a modified psychoanalytic approach. Neither of these ways of being a psychotherapist, of trying to help a person live his life more effectively, worked for me. In fact, when I was faced by someone who behaved toward me like a client-centered counselor or a psychoanalyst, it would almost make me vomit because it seemed inauthentic.

The nondirective school of therapy is relatively new. Let's see what the old school therapists would say in response to the client's question.

The Classic Freudian: "It is typical during this phase of therapy that the analyzee wants a more intimate relationship with their analyst. The Oedipal overtones are apparent in your languaging. Notice you said the equivalent of, 'You show me yours and I'll show you mine,'" says the scared analyst as his mind wanders to whether he has paid his sexual malpractice insurance or not. So you fire him and visit a Gestalt analyst.

The Gestalt Approach: "That's a great thing to work on today. Here now, imagine I'm sitting in this empty chair and I'm expressing my feelings and vulnerability to you. Feel into it. What would it look like, sound like. Don't be afraid to lash out, remember it's good to let bad feelings out," smiles the intern who has recently decided to call himself Fritz and wear a string of pearls, as a tribute to the master. So you end up verbally abusing yourself through the role of your own therapist and paying him to watch, a sort of voyeur's fee.

Another danger comes when a client has sunk into a funk. Some therapists try to get their clients out of that mood and become annoyed when the client continues to think in a way that the therapist fears is supporting the funk. These therapists get mad and in a very calm medical-science voice explain to their clients that they are "in denial," "being resistant," or "playing victim." Have you ever heard of anyone being told that they are playing victim and suddenly they find their power and start taking responsibility for their lives? Have you ever heard any person tell another that they are "in denial" and then suddenly that person gets a far-away "Aha!" look in his eyes? Followed by him saying, "Ah yes, now I see, it's really hurting little Bobby to be robbing his piggy bank on a weekly basis. I need to give up alcohol, smoking, gambling, wife-beating and overeating and dedicate my life to the selfless service of others!"

The therapist doesn't even have to tell her client that he is "in denial" or "being resistant." All the therapist needs to do is think in such terms and she will begin to convey the message through her jackal eyes. She will begin to have a certain detached, scientific, examining-a-bug-under-a-microscope attitude, which protects the therapist from feeling her own helplessness or sense of inadequacy. And God forbid that the client should comment on the message being sent. A friend of mine made the mistake of asking her therapist if he was feeling angry, to which the therapist replied, "So you feel that I am angry." And then he sat back in his white laboratory-coat silence, and stared with his jackal eyes to see what his guinea pig client would do with that one.

What a wonderfully safe business is psychotherapy. What other business do you know of where if the customer does not benefit or is unhappy, you get to blame the customer. That's ingenious! It would be like a car mechanic having a customer complain that his car still doesn't work. So the mechanic convinces the customer that he has a driving problem. Maybe he has one of the autoimmune diseases like driver's resistance, or ADD (auto driving disorder)?

If you are a therapist who wants to insure avoiding an authentic encounter with your client, it is important to understand the basic principles involved in preventing contact. It's actually simple. You just stay in your rational, thinking head, and away from places where you might actually with your client. Definitely stay far away from expressing anything that might be construed as a feeling or anything from your heart area. (It is similar to the ethical guidelines therapists are given. They are discouraged from going places like parties or intimate gatherings if they suspect a client might be there. This way they insure that their clients never actually meet them in a real-life setting.)

> -§-
> I want to speak to you from my need to connect, instead of using my words as a way to protect.
> -§-

In a rather typical outburst of irreverence, author Sidney Jourard once told his colleagues why they generated little true trust or respect from their clients: "In the first place, we do not let our clients know us as we really are; we regard that as nonprofessional conduct. If you look at us, you see many of us are fat, lifeless, constipated victims of the occupational diseases that come from a sedentary life."

The ineffectiveness of this attitude, of hiding behind a professional mask, was discovered very personally by Sidney Jourard as he began to do psychotherapeutic work while still in graduate school at Emory University. He began working with ordinary people in rural Georgia and found that his training handicapped him. I quote again from his book *The Transparent Self:*

> Through trial and error I found that if I abandoned my psychotherapeutic techniques and presented myself as a fairly intelligent, well-intentioned human being, if I shared some of my experience with problems similar to the ones that my patients were wrestling with, we got a good working relationship going. This was quite a departure from the orthodox techniques in which I had trained, and I felt anxious about it. But my research in self-disclosure was showing that disclosure invites or begets disclosure. My changes in psychotherapeutic behavior confirmed this. There is no way to force somebody to talk about himself. You can only invite.

Another tip for therapists striving for a certain inauthenticity is to think in terms of what the client "is" or what mental state she "is in." For example, the therapist can identify the client as a "food addict" or as being in a state of depression. He never wants to feel or say, "I am scared about how large you are becoming." He never wants to notice or express that, "I am frustrated with how often you shoot down exciting ideas before even trying them." This way he will stay safely cloistered away in the ivory tower of his role as therapist. The only thing more astonishing than how inappropriate the mental health community considers a therapist's crying or sharing his own feelings, is how healing it can be for the client.

-§-
I feel so helpless when you won't take your power back.
-§-

Martin Buber, the great Jewish mystic, told the father of Humanistic psychotherapy, Carl Rogers: "You can't do therapy as a therapist." I believe Buber was saying that, as long as you are playing therapist, thinking that you have more right to change your client than he has to change you, and that you know more than he does, you will be avoiding a more eye-to-eye, I and Thou encounter. It is only in the meeting, the blending of the psychic chemistries of two people, that the alchemy of transformation occurs. Jung referred to it as the exchange of psychic material.

I once got to speak with Rollo May as I was in training to be a therapist. I told him about my self doubts related to my childhood wounds. The great psychotherapist, told me, "The best therapists are the ones who have been wounded and are passionately working on their own healing process."

Dr. Laura Schlessinger is an example of a therapist (actually her doctorate is in another discipline) who never leaves her role and seldom empathizes with her clients if they have a political viewpoint different from hers. She gets totally flustered about ten times per show and accuses the caller of "playing stupid" or "playing victim." Her cure-all advice is "Get a life!" said with anger and conviction. This of course immediately enlightens and empowers all her thousands of callers who are starting to raise the planetary consciousness and lead the world into the new millennium.

With all this sarcasm you might think I was jealous of Dr. Laura. Well, maybe a little jealous of the number of people she is able to reach with her message, but not of her day-to-day experience. I am confident that anyone who so frequently thinks in those kinds of judgmental terms toward others is even harsher on themselves. Some evidence of that was a TV show about her. Some of the people who produce her radio show described her as a "perfectionist," which can be a polite euphemism for someone with a lot of self-hate and judgment.

I wish all of us therapists would own our self-hate and judgment instead of projecting it onto our clients through the sneaky, socially sanctioned ways that we do. For example, if the client says something that triggers anger in the therapist, the client is being aggressively provocative. If the therapist says something that triggers anger for client, the client is being defensive. If the client says something that the therapist doesn't understand, the client is being vague, incoherent and making loose associations. If the therapist says something that the client doesn't understand, the client is being resistant to therapy.

Some New Age therapists teach their clients how to be their own spin doctors, turning negatives into positives. When the client thinks, "Gosh, I'm depressed," they are taught by therapists to "reframe that" into, "All things work together for the universal good." It's too bad you cannot sue for "metaphysical malpractice." To me this is like seeing the red warning lights on your car dash and training yourself to imagine that it's really a Christmas tree light. Mechanics call these "idiot lights" because they are an ultimately simple indication that your car needs something you neglected to give it, like oil, and because if you can't figure out what the light means you'll soon be walking. One New Age therapist friend of mine was having his peace disturbed by the red light that appeared on his dashboard. He located a Band-Aid in his glove box, and covered the pesky distraction without even having to stop his car. How clever!

The Myth and Metaphor of "Mental Illness"

The whole concept of mental illness was invented in the mid-nineteenth century. Freud was beginning to discover that there was a lot of incest going on that explained much of the hysterical behavior of many women, particularly among family members of the Royal Academy of Medicine. He started to expose it, but then the academy freaked out and started threatening to kick him out. He basically recanted, and said that the hysterical behavior of these women is caused by this "mental illness" called conversion hysteria. This became the prototype for a whole class of diseases that launched the mental health field. This definition of certain behavior as a mental illness was something new. Up until that time an "illness" meant a bodily disorder.

Mental illness is a misnomer, because the mind does not get ill. The brain can become diseased or infected with viruses. But the mind does not develop diabetes, catch a cold, or become infected with HIV. What is called "mental illness" is often an adaptive strategy of thinking and behaving to cope with a will-breaking, crazy-making and soul-suppressing family and social system.

Psychiatrist Thomas Szasz, M.D., author of *The Myth of Mental Illness,* says:

> In modern medicine new diseases were discovered, in modern psychiatry they were invented. Persons who complained of pains and paralyses but were apparently physically intact in their bodies—that is, were healthy, by the old standards—were now declared to be suffering from a "functional illness." Mentally sick persons did not "will" their pathological behavior and were therefore considered "not responsible" for it.

What is funny is that even people who are discovered to be deliberately pretending to be ill—faking it, malingering—have been declared by modern psychiatry to be suffering from a mental illness, thereby absolving them of any responsibility for their choices. Just as Marx explained all human behavior as being caused by economic conditions in the society, Freud and most modern behaviorists have reduced human beings to puppets of family historical causes, or so-called "genetic-psychological" circumstances. Szasz takes exception to this because of the powerful effect that self-fulfilling prophetic diagnoses have on people. He wishes instead, as I do, to empower people: "I wish only to maximize the scope of voluntaristic explanations—in other words, to reintroduce freedom, choice, and responsibility into the conceptual framework and vocabulary of psychiatry."

So how do therapists and psychiatrists become attracted to participating in a system that denies personal responsibility? How do they come to support a caste system, where one group holds power by negatively labeling the other groups, reducing them to a subservient role?

To answer this question, we need to look at the some of the dynamics that are involved when people are abused or violated in some way. One of the strategies a victim of abuse often takes is to identify with the aggressor. So instead of identifying with the role of the weak, inferior victim of a physical or psychological domination in their childhood, they identify with the role of the strong, superior perpetrator.

A part of this superiority is a self-image of being caring, "nice" and meting out their medicine "for the patient's own good." A therapist with this image is no longer forced to meekly submit to the disciplinary diatribes of patriarchal parents. The therapist is now giving the lectures, in the form of penetrating analysis of, and helpful advice to, their childlike clients. They are no longer the powerless victims of a system of psycho-emotional domination. They are the commanding officers within a terribly powerful system that keeps the powers that be the powers that be. Many therapists have not fully felt and worked through their inevitable anger toward parents stuck in the prevailing paradigm of punishment and reward. Because of this they cannot be deeply empathic to the anger their patients have toward their parents. Without this deep empathy, their patients are stuck in an endless cycle of pain, self-hate and confusion.

Therapists who give their clients labels for themselves, or others, are providing them with a sort of lifejacket that may in the short run prevent them from drowning in shame and confusion. But just as lifejackets prevent you from going underneath the surface of the water, psychological labels can keep you on the surface of your consciousness, never diving deeper into the feelings and issues deeper in your body.

It is flowery license to abnegate responsibility for your thoughts and actions by indulging in "diagnostic denial." Can you imagine the Boston Strangler telling the judge, "I could not help it. I am a certified sociopathic serial killer"? Instead of feeling our painful feelings, or getting conscious of the distorted beliefs generating our destructive behaviors, we are taught to control ourselves by thinking about the behaviors. Instead of going within to come to "know thyself," we are offered a one-word explanation. I had a client once who also saw a psychiatrist to prescribe medication. He would become irate if I questioned his psychiatrist's theory that he was bipolar, caused by a chemical imbalance in his brain. When I suggested that the lack of endorphins in his brain might be the result of a certain type of thinking, the psychiatrist said he was going to report me to my licensing agency for violating professional ethics by trying to interfere with his patient's medical treatment.

Understanding the Needs Beneath the Deeds

A friend, Sara, told me that recently that she was about to attend a dance party with new friends. As she started looking for something to wear, she noticed a strong urge to go to the kitchen and grab a box of Oreos stashed in the kitchen cabinet behind the bag of brown rice. She started thinking about the label her therapist had recently given her: "Eating Disordered." She started thinking about how it was caused by her father's alcoholism, which allowed her to shift some of the shame and guilt onto him, through blame. Although the blame felt better than the shame, Sara was still left with angry feelings and an urge to stuff the anger down with food.

It was only much later that she was able to come out of her head, away from the righteous, therapeutically-supported blame and anger, and back into her body. It took the help of a friend who knew it would not be helpful to collude with her labels for herself or her father, and gave her high octane empathy instead. By high octane empathy, I mean that Sara's friend stayed emotionally fully present as Sara expressed first her anger, and then her hurt, sorrow, shame and grief. The word collusion can be read as "co-illusion" when it refers to people who reinforce our illusory labels.

As Sara came back into her body, she noticed that she was sad about not getting a certain quality of listening, acceptance, and attention from her father. She also became aware that she had been triggered by the thought "finding something to wear for the party." Sara identified that she was fearful about picking the right clothes to win attention and acceptance from her friends. She had unconsciously covered over this fear with a compulsive thought about eating Oreos.

Her attempt to understand her compulsive urge was not helped by what her therapist had offered her to think, that she had an "eating disorder." In fact it contributed to her confusion by keeping her up in her head. When she finally got back down into her body and emotions, she became aware that she was scared about not getting acceptance. She needed comfort and support. Becoming conscious of her basic need allowed her to see more options and feel more at choice. She could still choose Oreos, or she could find comfort through self-empathy, or empathy from others in the form of a reassuring phone call and/or hugs.

Sara's therapist was probably not able to really listen to Sara's feelings that were being expressed through her eating behavior. Even *beginning* to empathize with Sara's anger about not being listened to could make the therapist aware of his own anger about not being heard by his own parents. It is terrifying to be angry at powerful or punitive parents. Parents are literally a child's lifeline and their love line.

This fear of becoming angry with or questioning the patriarchal "powers that were" (their parents) or the "powers that be" (their licensing boards, college professors and professional associations), prevents therapists from being fully present. They have a particularly difficult time when someone is expressing the growing pains and angers that invariably come when people are breaking free from Dominator systems of thinking.

Alice Miller, the internationally renowned author, writes that only certain therapists have learned how to overcome their fear of expressing negative feelings to dysfunctional authority figures. Only these therapists, who have successfully resolved their own inner conflicts related to authority, can help their clients reach the emotional and intellectual freedom to become powerful, congruent and authentic. In the following quote, from her book *The Truth Will Set You Free,* she suggests that the underlying cause of anorexia is an inability to find someone to confide in. I would take her comments a step further and argue that most so-called "mental illnesses" have at their root a psyche that was never given what I would call our greatest psychological need: understanding.

What triggers anorexia in the first place is the tragedy of a young person unable to confide in anyone about her own feelings, to talk with anyone about how she needed to be nurtured as a child. Now she is unable, without help, to grasp the conflicts raging within her. In medical or psychiatric therapy she then encounters specialists equally concerned to evade such conflicts in themselves for fear that they might end up blaming their own parents. How can they hope to offer support to these young people? The patients can only summon the courage to put their discontent, their pain, their disappointment, their rage, and above all their needs into words if they are encouraged to do so by someone who does not share those fears or who has already experienced them and recognized them for what they are. There can be no doubt that successful therapeutic activity hinges on the therapist's own emotional development. The help provided by therapists, doctors, and social workers would take on a new dimension if knowledge of this childhood factor were widespread. So far, however, it appears to be taboo for the medical (and mental health) world.

A Culture of Compulsive Conformity

Sidney Jourard did research among the Psychology Department faculty at Emory University and found an interesting and significant correlation: "The more morally indignant the people were toward offbeat behavior, the less they criticized their parents and the more they glorified them." I believe this accounts for the subtle, cool, superior diagnostic disdain that many therapists carry for their "odd, dysfunctional" patients. Having never been taught to think outside the box of diagnostic labels, they see themselves as above, and removed from having a nurturing human relationship with the people who come to see them.

As long as a therapist has a fear of bucking the system or questioning the authority of his parents, his HMO, or of his school of psychological training, he can have no spiritual clarity about his intent in relating to his client. Without clear values it is easy to become an agent of the status quo. As a newly graduated therapist working at the residential treatment center for adolescents called The House of Hope, I experienced tremendous pressure to use techniques like withholding food. In order to inspire cooperation, kids were told they would not be allowed to see their parents. Heavy medications were prescribed for them in an effort to make them more manageable in the classroom. All this made me wonder what I was doing there.

The House of Hope was a small, family-owned operation. The most "respected" counselor carried a huge Smith and Wesson forty-five caliber pistol. The residents were all boys who had been in kiddy prison for everything from murder, rape, and armed robbery, to tagging (graffiti), and were now reentering society through the House of Hope. In the many months I was there, I must have seen a thousand incidents where the boys' behavior escalated to the point of throwing their schoolbooks, punching the walls, or hitting each other.

-§-
Client:
"Hey Doc, I can't sleep at night."
Therapist:
"You're an insomniac."
Client:
"Great! Now that I know what I am, I can sleep at night."
Therapist:
"That will be $185 please."
-§-

Some of the counselors had been working there for twenty years. It was these veteran counselors I found so amazing and amusing. They invariably picked the same intervention, and it always produced the same result. These models of experience and counseling wisdom would scream, "Calm down, cool out, take a chill pill," which most of the boys were already popping, prescribed by their psychiatrist. And the result of this intervention was perfectly consistent. The boys would yell louder, punch harder, and finding more dangerous things to throw. Ah, but at the House of Hope, hope springs eternal, even if nothing changes.

Most of the time allotted to treatment planning consisted of complaining about the stubbornness, defiance, or manipulativeness of their adolescent clients, saying things like, "That boy really is a slow learner." The therapists with the bigger degrees would say, "This boy is the clearest case of ADD I have seen." There is even a diagnosis for someone who refuses to obey another's orders: Oppositional Defiant

Disorder. It was another label for, "kids whose wills we haven't yet figured out how to break."

Week after week the therapists would come up with the same "interventions," a fancy clinical word for "strategies to manipulate behavior." These interventions were just variations on the same theme of punishments and rewards, designed to prepare the children to live in the "real world" of a coercive culture.

Social Conformity

What is the purpose of the "helping professions?" For a psychiatrist it is sadly simplistic: to cure someone's "mental illness." For the behavioral psychologist: to correct a "dysfunctional behavior." The accepted purpose of psychotherapy in our culture has been aptly described by Jourard in the following way:

> Up to the present, psychotherapists have functioned as emergency socialization agents; their job has been to correct the failures of family, school, and other socialization agencies to "shape up" a citizen so his behavior would not be a problem to everyone else. People who did not "fit" were designated mentally ill. An entire mythology of illness and its cure was gradually evolved by the medical profession, and no psychotherapist was unaffected by this ideology. Psychologists, clergymen, social workers, and counselors of all kinds were trained to view misfitting people as sufferers from "mental disease," and they were led to believe that if they mastered certain theories and techniques for transacting with Them, the patients, they would effect a cure. From this view people who want to make love, not war, are seen as impractical, schizoid, or seditious.

One of my personal challenges in working with the people who come to see me is to be aware of the "politics of psychotherapy." I need to be careful not to invalidate the experience of those who find living in our culture intolerable. I need to be careful not to try to help anyone become "normal" in the name of "treatment."

Instead I want the challenge of interacting authentically with the people who come to see me, and living my life in such an authentic way that I inspire courage on the part of others to do the same. This can keep me from getting caught in the trap of what Jourard called "the manipulative medical model." Instead my focus on authenticity can help me lead by example of a courageous, creative, unique expression of *me*. As I do this I am no longer a "nice" respected member of my profession in this culture, but instead someone who endeavors to support others in finding their authentic path. The last thing I want is followers on my path. If I do get followers then I am leading them astray, and therefore will chase them away to find their own path. For my path is mine alone and yours is yours alone.

Is a therapist's license a license to judge, with socially sanctioned labels? Are these labels okay, because you've been trained in their scientific use? For the therapist, "Sex Addict" might equal someone whose sexual values differ from the therapist's. For the conservative fundamentalist religious therapist, "Sex Addict" might equal anyone who masturbates, is gay, has premarital sex, has sex with more than one person, uses any sexual aids, has AIDS, has sex other than in the supine position, has sex with the lights on, or anyone who laughs at the following joke:

Do you know why Santa is so jolly?

Because he knows where all the bad girls live.

William Whyte in his *Organization Man* warned us that modern man's enemies may turn out to be a "mild-looking group of therapists, who would be doing what they did to help you." He was referring to the tendency to use social sciences in support of the social ethic of our historical period; thus the process of helping people may actually make them conformist and tend toward the destruction of individuality.

Jean Houston, prolific author and past president of the Association of Humanistic Psychology, once told me, "Diagnoses are the character assassination of psychiatrists." Albert Einstein had all the symptoms of a profound, severe case of Attention Deficit Disorder. He didn't speak until he was four and didn't read until he was seven. Thank God they didn't have such an advanced diagnosis and treatment back then. What if some well-intentioned social worker had gotten him some prescription medication to help him fit in better? It may have stunted his development, or worse—robbed the world of his genius. I am reminded of all the recent national news stories about a link they are now finding between prescription psychiatric medications and suicides in children.

Dr. Marshall Rosenberg who is himself a clinical psychologist, tells this joke at many of his trainings: "Growing up in Detroit I learned a rather crude, unsophisticated dialect of jackal language. If someone cut me off in traffic, I might stick my head out the window and scream 'You idiot!' on a good day. But now that I have my Ph.D. and a license to do psychotherapy on people, I am much more refined. Now I would say 'You pseudoneurotic schizophrenic with borderline tendencies!'" And with that Marshall breaks out his guitar and sings:

The Sink or Shrink Blues
by Marshall Rosenberg

I went to a shrink in a clinic near me.
He said, I was a case of total pathology.
I said, "Shrink, I knew that before I came in.
I need someone to care, not this analyzin'."
He asked me if I had any strange habits.
I said, "A few, but I'm always willing to learn some more."
So he gave me some pills and said to take some each day.
I said, "Shrink, pills won't take my blues away.
My blues come from people like you
Who know what I am, but not what I've been through."
You see folks, he was one of those old fashioned doctors.
He still thought you needed a prescription to get drugs.
Well that shrink saw what he was trained to see.
He just never got around to seeing me.
So I left that shrink; I wasn't impressed.
Now there's two who flew that cuckoo's nest.

Signs of a Nice Therapist

One client's lament: "There was a real person behind my last counselor. Too bad I never got to know her." A more helpful therapist might be a real person who shows up with her presence in the form of empathy and honesty — not empty reflective listening, theorizing, analyzing, and advice-giving. And there is a difference between empathizing and psychologizing. Make sure you choose a therapist who knows the difference. Nice therapists psychologize, real therapists empathize, and offer vulnerable honesty.

Six warning signs that you are with a nice therapist:

1. (In Hollywood, the great ego village of California): You complain to your therapist that you are depressed because you think you are ugly and she says, "Have you considered cosmetic surgery?"

2. He never interrupts you even if you are an Energizer Bunny Babbleonian.

3. She smiles broadly as she tells you your boyfriend fits the profile of a sociopathic stalker.

4. When you tell him that your own dog bit you, your truck broke down and your girlfriend left, he asks in the kindest, sweetest tone: "Why are you creating this in your life?" Then when your rage comes up in response, you feel like a madman in comparison to this gentle, helpful, enlightened soul.

5. You say that your boyfriend sometimes forgets to knock before entering your room, and she suggest a restraining order.

6. You tell your therapist he is an aloof, distant, intellectualizing talking head. He replies, "When did you first start feeling this way?"

If you yourself are a therapist and want to see if you fit into my diagnosis of "niceneck" therapist consider the following criteria. You just might be a "niceneck" therapist if:

1. You start purposely looking at your watch when you are bored with certain clients.

2. You consume more Prozac than your whole clientele put together.

3. If, more than once a week, you wake up in the middle of the night screaming, "I'm not your father!"

4. Diagnosing your clients gives you a rush of superiority while still allowing you to believe you are being compassionate.

5. You are forever thinking your clients should be making more progress than they are.

6. You think you "should" be empathetic toward your patients.

I am not saying that all therapists are "nicenecks." I believe that more and more therapists are developing their presence and skill—even a couple of psychiatrists! It is less likely that these more conscious therapists will be found submitting to the Dominator organizational systems of an HMO, PPO, or government agency. They are much more likely to be found in private or a small group practice. You will know you have found a conscious therapist if:

1. You leave the session feeling truly heard.

2. The therapist shares his own emotions in the session.

3. She interrupts you when you are babbling on.

4. What she says matches her facial expression. She doesn't smile as she says, "You were late for your appointment again."

5. People in your community have good things to say about her.

6. She is not a behaviorist, not big on medications, does not use labels for your situation or condition, and does not wear polyester pantsuits.

7. She does not try to cram your life history into her school of thought or psychological theory.

8. She is willing to allow you to interview her as thoroughly and deeply as you want.

Such a therapist is willing to meet you in a soul-to-soul meeting, without any roles in between. In Virginia Satir's book *The Use of Self in Therapy,* she describes how powerful and healing it is for a therapist to bring her total self, her voice, her body, her emotions, her experience into an authentic encounter with the client. Such a thera-pist is not nice; she is real.

Chapter

OUR CULTURE DOESN'T WORK ANYMORE

Now that I'm all worked up, I'm going to stop being nice and tell you what I really think about our culture. I think the dying sociologist Morrie Schwartz described my views accurately when he told ABC newsman Ted Koppel, "Our culture does not work any more. We need to create a new one!"

How sad that so many of us well-intentioned, "nice" people have sat by and watched this become a domination culture. Domination cultures only occur because submissive people have permitted it to happen.

And what is a domination culture? A domination culture organizes itself so that a few dominate the many. Therefore it is basically anti-democratic. It does not value the equality or importance of the individual, as reflected in the democratic value of one person—one vote. These anti-democratic values are seen in the family system structures where parents (usually the father) proclaim to have the best, or God-given, judgment and so makes the rules for everyone, and wears the pants in the family. On the societal level, in the vast majority of our schools, businesses, churches, and government, the leaders use coercive punishments and rewards to impose the will of the few on the many, but of course only "for their own good."

If we're going to create a new culture, as Morrie suggested, we will have to let our children know the truth about the culture we live in. We need to tell them, for example, that if you murder someone and you are wealthy, you are much, much more likely to go free than if you are poor. If you're convicted, you are much more likely to get a death sentence if you are African American or Hispanic, and a life sentence if you are Caucasian. If you are female, you will likely get paid less for whatever you do than if you are male. We are going to have to admit to our children that really we are a cast system disguised as a democracy.

Openness and honesty about the larger culture we live in is just one small thread in a tapestry of transparency that I would like to see develop in our culture. The most nurturing transparency occurs within the community of our circle of friends. However, you may have noticed that many of our little community cultures are less than open, honest and nurturing to their members. Instead they are whirlpools of gossip, backbiting, infighting and politicking.

The Myth That Honesty Hurts or Harms

One of the pillars in the paradigm of a culture of cruelty is this belief: expressing oneself honestly causes psychological pain for others.

Parents are taught to tell their children, "It hurts Mommy's feelings when you tell her that the dinner she slaved over a hot stove to make, 'sucks'." Best-selling American parenting books unwittingly teach parents how to set these kinds of guilt hooks deep into their children's hearts. Then emotional manipulation can be effectively used to control feelings and behavior through the use of fear, guilt and shame. It is not the intention of these parenting gurus to harm children. From their perspective they are disciplining and preparing the children for the "real world." But we must be very careful of preparing children to fit into organizations like certain soulless corporations, armies, governments and schools that do not honor an individual's autonomy and spirit.

One key to transforming this familiar family scene is to tell the truth. The kids did not hurt Mommy. What hurt was what she said to herself. A more self-aware mommy might notice that her hurt is coming from her interpretation of the child's honesty as a rejection of her. If the child is under nine, she would choose to deal with her feelings by asking her husband or a friend for empathy about what was triggered, or do some journaling. She might say to herself, "I'm angry because I'm thinking children should hide their dissatisfaction." Or she might say, "I'm feeling hurt because I think my child does not care about my feelings," or, "I'm ashamed that maybe I am a poor cook," or, "I feel guilty because I think I should have realized I was over-salting the food."

-§-
Relationships are not fair or unfair, they are a mystery to be patiently, persistently, passionately unwrapped.
-§-

If the child is mature enough to understand, the Mommy might tell the child, "I hear you do not like the food. Would you acknowledge, though, that I did try hard to make you some food you like?"

Self-awareness is just that simple. No deep insight or analysis is required. Yet most of us lack this simple skill. Instead, we habitually blame, punish, and project. Or we terribly nice people smile and pretend that we are not bleeding internally. Sadly, these patterns of dishonesty destroy transparency and congruency. When we are transparent, we are honest and self-responsible. We express what is alive and truly going on within us. We are congruent when we say what we are feeling—and our face, gesture and tone are all in concert with that feeling.

If I am incongruent, you will instantly sense I am not trustworthy. You will withhold cooperation. Trust is the basic factor needed for cooperation. When we trust, we open our eyes to another's humanness. Trust lets us empathize. It allows for natural openness and affection. It clarifies our understanding of each other. Trust allows for the free flow of honesty, accurate perceptions of each other, risk-taking and love. In cultures and couples where this basic trust is missing, the need arises for a great degree of external control. That means rules, agreements, commitments, policing, punishment and a general loss of freedom. True freedom is not the freedom to own three SUV's and a super-wide-screen TV, but a joyful flow of connectedness, peace and creativity within one's community. When a group or a couple has transparency, a full disclosure of all the important elements of one's inner and outer life, then individuals cannot be turned against each other through the spread of false rumors. I once started a group like this of twenty six "Love Pioneers." In this close knit tribe that we created to provide community support for our relationship, we had an interesting confidentiality agreement. It went like this: "You can be confident that if it is juicy we are going to share it with the whole tribe. We did not have a problem with factions, gossip or false rumors because we all knew the truth about what was going on with each other on every level. This allows trust to grow. The commitment to stay open to each other even when someone does something out of integrity makes it much easier for everyone to keep telling the whole truth. Therefore we must stop punishing people not only for telling the truth, but we must stop punishing altogether, if we are to develop a truthful group, family or couple.

Part of the reason most of us do not have this true freedom is because we live in what I call the a soap opera culture of the Five C's. Collision, Collusion, Confusion, Cover-up, and Chicken Soup. Our personal communities stay superficial, or knotted up in strife and pain-filled struggle, because we do not know how to support each other in working through the difficulties that inevitably come up with each other. We can have deep intimacy only if we have strong skills at working through the inevitable conflicts that arise as human beings interact closely.

The fear that is generated by coping with conflict using the Five C's severely limits tolerance of mistake-making and, therefore, growth and creative individual expression. This contributes to divisiveness in the community, which frequently results in schisms and conflicting camps. Look at the cliques in high schools. It was the venom between some of these cliques that led to several different school shootings, including Columbine.

It is also painful, isolating and depressing to stuff down pain to protect another person's reputation in the community (Cover-up). Thinking that you are undermining someone's respect within their community can lead to debilitating guilt. It is this guilt and the fear of this guilt that prevents an open, free flow of communication within a community. This constipation of communication creates all kinds of violent, unhealthy, painful consequences for that community, including scape-goating, low enthusiasm, and power struggles.

Because we have so few true forums for transparency in our personal communities, honesty gets repressed, split off and closed up. Any time any part of ourselves, whether it be sadness, anger, fear or sexuality, gets separated or shut down, it begins to take on a demonic life of its own, and usually comes out in a destructive way. Then, according to Virginia Satir, "they become like ravenous dogs that you put down in the basement. And one day when you least expect it, they bust the door down and wreak havoc." In community, when honesty is not given its space, gossip and in-fighting will soon take its place.

Because we live in a punishment/reward, patriarchal, and often judgmental culture, it can be quite dangerous to be honest about what is happening. Consider the cost Martin Luther King, Jr. (and Jesus) paid for telling it like it is. However, if we do not run the risk of telling the whole truth, we set in motion inescapable dynamics destructive to harmony among human beings. These destructive dynamics occur based on a principle of ecology that says, "Nature hates a closed system."

Transparency Sets You Free

Dieter Duhm, the founder of the Zegg Community in Germany, (Zegg stands for a German phrase which means "an experiment in cultural design.") says that it is particularly important to keep communication open and flowing in those areas we tend to have shame around and are tempted to sweep under the rug. These things include sex, anger, fear, disease and money.

Duhm wrote:

Building a humane community usually means confronting difficulties that are deeply rooted in people. Instead of the fixation on humanitarian slogans and demands, what is needed is that emotional reality must at all times and places be made visible, with as playful and joyful methods as possible, until all pretense and hypocrisy drop away. Try to make what happens in the community understandable and transparent to everyone, especially emotional and sexual processes, for they are behind almost everything that makes the group situation difficult and opaque. Only if all processes are transparent will the members lose their paranoia, and the destructive processes will be kept from leading a life of their own. Only then can the causes of rifts and fractures in the group be treated before it is too late.

It Takes a Village to Raise a Relationship

It is particularly difficult for couples to thrive in a healthy way in the culture common to most American communities. When one party of the couple reaches out to the community for understanding about some pain or struggle she is having with her partner, nine times out of ten, all she will get is collusion, collision, confusion, chicken soup or cover-up. Here's an example: A desperately-seeking-help Susan says to her girlfriend, "I am scared that my boyfriend is going to a party in hopes of seeing his former girlfriend." Here are some of the responses typical in a dysfunctional culture:

Collusion: "You're right, that is abusive. He needs a good therapist."

Collision: "Don't be so insecure. You will suffocate the man." This kind of collision can happen when the person you are sharing your feelings with has his own fear or pain triggered. Then instead of empathizing with you, he offers his own reaction, often in the form of a psychological diagnosis.

Confusion: "How could you even think that about him?"

Chicken Soup: "Have you considered cosmetic surgery?" (This is what a best girlfriend from Hollywood actually said to a friend after she confessed that her husband was starting to look at other women.)

Health Nut Chicken Soup: "You sound depressed. Zinc is very good for depression. Here, I think I have some here in my purse. I cannot find the zinc, but I did find this yummy Ginseng Protein Bar which should help balance some of that yucky yang energy you're feeling."

New Age Chicken Soup: "Why are you creating this in your life? Maybe you need to attend this seminar this weekend, with the Jolly Llama, called Totally Transforming Your Life."

Cover-up: "I am sure it's harmless. How could he think of leaving you for her? Have some bologna hors d'oeuvres."

Susan also may feel scared to tell her girlfriend the painful truth, for fear of judgment that she is needy or dependent—or the more sophisticated judgment, "codependent." And there is always the fear that her girlfriend will gossip in the community, telling others that she cannot keep her man happy. In many a competitive community, sharing this vulnerability will be perceived as a weakness in the relationship and therefore a potential opening for other women to try to steal him away.

Many women in our culture live in constant fear of competition, which creates an atmosphere of mistrust in the community of women. This mistrust creates shallowness of relating, which prevents women from drawing strength from their potential collective unity. When women do not have this strength that comes from their collective emotional unity, they feel weak, insecure, and vulnerable. When they bring this fear and emotional depletion to their male partners, the men sometimes feel overwhelmed and inadequate at not being able to meet their emotional needs. Men will

-§-
If I cannot tell you my "No," I am never really saying "Yes!" I am simply being swept along.
-§-

frequently deal with their overwhelm and inadequacy by either withdrawing or blaming. The blaming may sound like this: "You're so needy, overly sensitive, controlling, and demanding."

A key component in strong community is that the members support people in their strengths, instead of colluding with them in their powerlessness. When women are not in a primary relationship the power of their sisterhood is often much stronger. They are not so caught up in the fear of competition. This fear of competition includes fear of losing their partner to a girlfriend and fear of feeling shame when they compare themselves to that girlfriend unfavorably. Until a woman can develop a network of strong women, and has experience with empathy and emotional honesty, she will likely continue to create a sort of A-Frame dependency with her partners. This is where she perceives her partner's needs for spontaneity, freedom, involvement with the world and connection with others as abandonment, and he perceives her needs for closeness, security, continuity, and reassurance as controlling and needy. His slightest request for freedom triggers her fear of abandonment and comparison. Her slightest request for reassurance or security is judged by him as a weakness, a lack of trust in him or a demanding need to control. This of course is not a gender-rigid dynamic. I have seen gender roles reversed many times. Other polarizations within couples include closeness v. autonomy, security v. spontaneity, certainty v. uncertainty, and being trusted v. being valued.

Creating Intimate Community

How do we create intimacy in communities of men and women? One way is to lay our cards on the table about how we feel about each other's partners. What if the women just told each other who they were attracted to, and whether they planned to take action on this attraction. Maybe we would begin to create an atmosphere of trust where at least such things could be talked about before they were acted upon in secrecy. This could allow for dialogue between all the concerned parties—instead of the covert war of stealth and competition, which keeps us all talking about the weather and subconsciously looking for clues about who is hitting on whom. This atmosphere of trust is destroyed by the injunction not to talk about the inevitable attractions that take place between people. Most women have a strong intuitive sense about who is attracted to whom anyway. It is the attempt to hide this truth and cover it up that creates so much mistrust. Also without a clear expression of how people intend to act on or respond to these attractions, great fear is often generated as women and men try to protect themselves from the possible loss of the loved one.

Another reason couples need transparent community so much is to break up the polarization dynamic that so frequently occurs when two human beings engage each other deeply. Polarization within a couple is difficult to discharge without contact with outside positive and negative energies. I use the words positive and negative in an electrical or electromagnetic sense, not good or bad. Positive and negative poles of a magnet repel each other when brought into close contact, yet they are naturally and dynamically on opposite ends of the same magnet. So too with couples. As they are brought into close contact, opposites attract. Attraction and tension develop between the neatnicks and the slobs, the spendthrifts and the misers, the spontaneous and the cautious, the extroverts and the introverts, the freedom loving kites and the grounded strings, the party animals and the homebodies.

Two things are desperately needed if harmonious development of the relationship is to occur. One is good communication skills and the other is a mature outside support system. By outside, I mean other people in the community besides the dynamic duo themselves. By "positive" outside support I mean self-responsible honesty, and by "negative" I mean the vital vacuum force of empathy. This vacuum force sucks conflicts, anger, resentments, and withholds onto the table of discussion. It is created by people who have great presence, a non-judgmental attitude, an ability for accurate empathy, and great listening skills.

It is tragic to me that so many times an attempt to get help from an outside source is interpreted as a threat, betrayal, or an abandonment. Or sometimes it is interpreted as more proof that one is not enough, otherwise the partner would have no outside needs. Other tragic interpretations include:

1. "You're unwilling to work it out just between us."

2. "You're sharing this with others to spite me."

3. "We're admitting to our friends that our relationship has failed."

4. "This is the beginning of the end."

5. "You don't have faith in the relationship."

6. "It's disloyal to air the family's dirty laundry."

7. "You're telling others to get revenge on me."

In polarization, the woman's old wounds trigger the man's old wounds, and vice versa. (Of course these dynamics also occur in all types of relationships: gay, bisexual, multiple, and platonic.) There are thousands of nuances within these different examples. Part of the reason that we feel strong attractions to certain people is because of the concave and convex dovetailing of wounds. We are attracted to our opposite, to someone who has qualities we do not possess, the qualities that, as a pair, make us more whole. The male, yang quality is pulled toward the female, yin quality.

-§-
There are no men and women, only people with different plumage, plumbage and social programming.
-§-

An example of this would be where partner A has been wounded in the area of security. Perhaps one or both parents died or left or were not emotionally present. She is attracted to someone who seems to display a certain confidence or trust in life.

Partner B has been wounded in the area of freedom. His freedom was restricted or lost and there is a lingering fear that that freedom will be given away for the sake of the relationship. So the cycle begins:

She: "I am worried about you going to that party, because your ex girlfriend Jane is going to be there."

He: "Great! Now I have to get clearance before I can go anywhere just in case there are any known past lovers or felons around. Why don't you just get me one of those ankle bracelets that sound an alarm whenever I get more than fifty feet from the house? I feel like I am under house arrest and you are my parole officer."

Now why doesn't he just go ahead and assert his freedom needs? Why doesn't he just say, "Look, I really want to go to this party, and I trust you to deal with your fear and pain about it"? It is partly because of his underlying fear that if he does that, he will be abandoned. He also fears that his community will judge him as selfish and shun him. He could not give her any understanding for her fear because of his own reaction of fear about giving up his freedom again. She can not understand his need related to wanting to go to the party because her fear of abandonment and fear of comparison has been triggered.

How Jealousy Prevents Peace

There is another way of creating what I call "deep community." Duhm says that as long as one person's giving attention to, or caring for another, triggers pain in a third party, true community is difficult to establish. According to Duhm, this dynamic of jealousy or possessiveness is a primary reason groups and communities stay in almost constant covert or overt conflict. The other primary dynamic destructive to group harmony is repression of parts of ourselves, particularly our animal nature.

These conclusions were reached after a group of about fifty Germans set out to bring a teaching of nonviolence to Germany. For a number of years, as they tried to organize themselves to do this teaching, they found themselves constantly bickering, gossiping, and engaging each other in a politically painful way. It is no accident that these Germans see the desperate importance of preventing repression and its relationship to violence. German history is filled with decades of repression, followed by an explosion of the most hideous kind of violence. The catastrophic consequences of repression of our animal nature can even be predicted by those who deeply understand the workings of the collective unconscious. Carl Jung was such a man and predicted the coming of WWII. As we all know, wild animals in the wild are not that dangerous, until they are put in cages. It is the cage that drives the wild animal mad and turns it into the devouring demon of our nightmares. Carl Jung wrote that 'the blond beast' could be heard prowling in it's underground prison. It had become a beast due to centuries of repression created when "Christianity split the Germanic barbarian into an upper half and a lower half, and confined the lower to that underground prison."

It is fascinating to me that Jesus, the great peacemaker of Christianity, was born in a manger among the other animals. This newborn mammal is both animal and incarnation of God. Both beast and sacred. This is the bringing of the lower animal unconscious into the higher divine conscious that Jung said was the path to peace and elevated consciousness. This bringing together of the humble animal nature with the Christ consciousness made the angels sing of peace on earth.

Dr. Andrew Schmookler, summa cum laude graduate of Harvard, in his book *Out of Weakness* writes "Without such reconciliation, without this recognition of the indissoluble link between the natural and the sacred, the beast becomes demonized. It is a central insight of Jungian psychology that denial makes more sinister what is denied."

In order to prevent another cycle of this kind of repression and its resulting rage, a group of German peace pioneers decided they would first need to experience unrepressed consciousness of nonviolence themselves, before they could bring it to Germany. They decided to move in together on some land in the Black Forest to do the inner integration work needed to become nonviolent themselves. After ten years they began to gain insight into these most insidious dynamics of jealousy, repression and their sisters: greed, violence and revenge. They determined that these were the primary elements preventing harmony and deep connection within the community. As they developed processes (which they called "The Forum") to solve the problem of jealousy and repression, they began to become a very powerful and harmonious spiritual group. Today they work around the globe, including the Middle East, to help people see the connection between repression and violence, and build a bridge back to holy wholeness.

Over the centuries, peacemakers have gone to extreme lengths to try to solve the problem of human's inhumanity to humankind. On one level it seems obvious that greed, jealousy and possessiveness are the roots of violence. One solution I tried was the path of the celibate monk, which failed miserably for me. It did not integrate my whole body, which I needed to do, in order to be at peace. I tried to escape possessiveness by withdrawing from any relationship that might become possessive. But my problem with this was not about having no relationship; it was getting caught in the spirit of possessiveness. My motto in relationships had been, "You can have anything you want except your freedom." After way too many years, I left the ashram. I finally got the message that Ram Dass's spiritual guide, Emanuel, gave him: "You live in the school of the earth plane, why not take the curriculum?" A big part of this curriculum is about natural unconditional love, which is mutually exclusive with possessiveness. In a section of his book entitled "Beyond Possessiveness," Schmookler writes these words:

> As with material possession, so with sexual. In part, the celibacy of Christian (and some other) monks is evidence of a failure of their spiritual path to achieve peace with the body, an inability to incorporate the whole human being within the compass of spiritual harmony. But in part also the practice of celibacy expresses the spiritual understanding that it is important to learn not to hold on. The way of the monk, it seems to me, emerges as a reaction against the tendency of the man of war, and as the one is extreme in one way, the other goes to the opposite extreme. The monk rejects this world, which is corrupted by the warrior's spirit, saying that our true life is in another realm altogether. But I believe that it is to this world we are born, and in relation to this world that our true fulfillment and true calling are to be found.

In order to answer this true calling we need strong, supportive, nurturing relationships. And until there is deep, strong community that supports autonomy, unconditional love and a non-repressive sexuality, it is very difficult to sustain deep, alive, creative relationships. The fact that someone has had a reaction to one person giving attention, recognition, affection to a third person is seldom talked about in most communities. And of course it happens even when there is no romantic interest involved at all. Jealousy and possessiveness can and does occur across all gender, orientation and relationship lines. Wherever three or more of us are gathered in the name of relating, jealousy can emerge. And it frequently does, although it may be difficult to detect because people have so much shame about it that they usually hide it very well.

Jealousy can be found among the most sophisticated and highly educated people and is far, far more rampant and influential than I ever perceived before I began to study it. Here's what well-known author and public TV guru Wayne Dyer says about the pervasiveness of jealousy:

> Most of you are jealous and possessive in your love. When your love turns to possessiveness it makes demands. The demands then alienate the loved one and you incorporate anger and fear into the relationship. With these come bitterness and aggression, and whether we speak of individual love relationships or global interactions, what you call love, but is in fact ownership and manipulation, takes over and the problems then flow.

There are many reasons why a community does not meet the needs of its members for healthy relationships and stays in what M. Scott Peck, MD, calls the superficial phase of pseudomutuality. A healthy community is like a lapidary's rock tumblers. You put in a pile of rocks and tumble them until they are shiny and smooth. Polite and nice communities are like putting a bunch of marshmallows in the tumbler. In the end they come out just the same. Here are a few dynamics and beliefs that keep nice, superficial communities ever exploring new depths in shallowness:

1. The community members are unconsciously afraid of triggering each other's jealousy so they stay away from really making contact with another.

2. There is little knowledge of how to work through jealousy if it does arise in oneself.

3. There is little knowledge of how to support others in working through jealousy if it arises in them.

4. Jealousy is supported as a proof of love.

If you don't think American pop culture values, supports, glamorizes and sexualizes jealousy, look at the June 2000 edition of *Psychology Today*. On the front cover in huge red letters you will read

Jealousy — why we need it as much as love and sex." The background picture is the sexy face of a young woman — with green eyes, of course. In the article inside, called "Prescription for Passion," Dr. David M. Buss, Ph.D., says, "Jealousy ignites rage, shame, even life-threatening violence. But it is just as necessary as love. In fact, it preserves and protects that fragile emotion. Consider it a kind of old-fashioned mate insurance, an evolutionary glue that holds modern couples together." He does "scientific" research in which he finds that successful women use jealousy to test the love in their relationship, suggesting that if there is no jealousy there is no love. And they confront commitment problems by inducing jealousy to correct "imbalances" — i.e., situations where she wants him more than he wants her.

5. If someone expresses caring or recognition to one person, it is assumed to mean they do not respect or care for the others in the group or the other member of a couple.

6. Doing favors or acts of caring creates a bank account of paybacks owed. These paybacks are due on demand. If not paid on demand, vicious gossip is spread. The value is, "If I really care about someone or have done a lot for them, they should give me whatever I want, whenever I want it."

7. There is a constant competition for status, airtime, attention, and recognition that is not consciously acknowledged or negotiated.

8. This "competition compulsion" ("Go Gators!") is partly cultural conditioning and partly a belief that if one person gets their need for attention met, there will be less for others. This is equivalent to

thinking that if I have health, there will be less health left over for the rest of the people in the world.

9. There is a fear of having intimate contact, even eye contact, with members of the opposite sex for fear of incurring an obligation to "go all the way."

Sex, Violence, and Religious Lies

What creates all this sense of scarcity and jealousy in our culture? One element is something of which we Americans are very proud, competition. Competition and jealousy go hand in hand. When we compete for grades in school, we are measuring ourselves, and our self-worth, in comparison to others. When we are gripped by jealousy, we see ourselves in a competition for love, and coming up short in comparison to the person of whom we are jealous. We are receiving a big fat F (as in failure) in "Loveability." With grades, there is a consciousness of artificial scarcity created, as if there are only so many A's in the teacher's grading pencil. When we are in jealousy, we are caught in a fearful fantasy that says there is only so much love to go around, and I am about to have my fair share taken from me.

We have all heard the horror stories about Little League parents who scream at their kids, each other and the umpires—or about high school kids who kill themselves after losing an important football game, or other competitive event. Recently in middle America, a hockey Dad was convicted of killing another hockey Dad with his bare hands. There is tremendous pressure to be the one and only one that comes out on top, the cheered winner instead of the jeered loser. Sadly, we bring this same pressure and fear of feeling "worth less" into our love life. We cannot simply coat check this "competition consciousness" at our bedroom door. We bring it into all our love relationships in this culture. When our beloved gets close to someone else, we feel we have lost at the game of love. If we are not in total control of our partner, or if she shares closeness with someone else, we are taught to interpret it as meaning that we are somehow inferior.

What do young men ask each other the day after the big date with the new girl at school? "Did you score? Did you take her?" As if love is a game, a big competition, where one person beats, bests and dominates another. These same young men are taught that intimacy is effeminate and real men win by getting to "home plate," a euphemism for sexual intercourse. This value of having sex without feelings is how many young men get initiated into "manhood." It is a raucous seedy sex scene with a prostitute and laughing fraternity brothers or military buddies standing by. On the other side, young women are taught that life is about surrendering into the romantic arms of a solitary Prince Charming. Men conquer, women cave in.

What are the roots of this domination/submission dynamic in our personal love relationships? Just like the fish in water, we do not see the culture we are immersed in. Here is an illustration from Riane Eisler's book *Sacred Pleasure*:

> We may not be conscious of it, but we have all been influenced in how we think of sex by what we have been taught about our sexual origins. Take for example the familiar cartoon of the club-carrying caveman dragging a woman around by her hair. In a few, "amusing" strokes it tells us that from time immemorial men have equated sex with violence and women have been passive sex objects. In other words, it teaches us that sex, male dominance, and violence are all of one cloth — and that underneath our veneer of civilization, this is how it is.

In another book by Eisler, *The Chalice and the Blade,* she explains how this male myth about the nature of our sexuality and mankind was created. She suggests that male archeologists and historians, who had already been socialized into stereotypical Western male gender roles, interpreted history through those glasses, and came out with a highly skewed picture of Paleolithic and Neolithic civilization. Like someone taking a Rorschach Ink Blot Test, they saw spears and weapons, where later interpretations indicated tree branches and plants. These scholars assumed that it was only men who painted. Today there is evidence that much of it was done by women. Where these male scholars saw bloodthirsty, warlike hunters, it is now evident that these earliest of paintings are of women dancing in circles. And, most importantly, the supposedly objective scientists saw "the insignificant expressions of a crude form of pornography:" male sex objects, painted by some horny cave boy graffiti artist. Subsequent historians have now made clear that these paintings and figurines are the symbolic representation of a female centered anthropomorphic form of worship of Gaia, the great Mother Goddess, Giver of All. They were tantric, Stone Age, spiritual ecologists. This art and many other artifacts, previously misunderstood, now reveal a Goddess-centered culture and social structure without images of male domination, war, or wide disparities in class (as shown by an equality of precious burial objects, art and money in male and female burial sites).

For tens of thousands of years men and women worked in equal partnership, with women as priestesses, leaders and heads of clans. There was no art glorifying weapons, battles, slavery or angry male deities like the thunderbolt-throwing Zeus. From studying the history of these artifacts, Eisler, (in the same book,) draws the following conclusion: "If the central religious image was a woman giving birth and not, as in our time, a man dying on a cross, it would not be unreasonable to infer that life and the love of life — rather than death and the fear of death — were dominant in society as well as art."

So although our culture has come to equate sex with domination and violence, it is interesting to note that it has not always been this way. It was a developmental direction that our Western civilization took, which great parts of ancient cultures, as described above, and other small lesser-known modern cultures did not. The historical development of the mythological figure of Cupid, the god of love, provides a microcosm of the process. He started out being not male, but androgynous in Paleolithic art. By Greek times he was not only the son of Aphrodite, the Greek goddess of love, but son of Aries, the Greek god of war. In early pictures he/she was a sweet, innocent, chubby cherub, but by Roman times he was the capricious, malicious winged little boy armed with bow and arrows. He was then also accompanied by Anteros, who avenged unrequited love. Perhaps he could be called the god of envy or jealousy. What started out as an image of feminine sexual creativity became a symbol of the insecure, jealous male conquering warrior.

With this shift came a political change. As the Roman Emperor Constantine hijacked Christianity, women, children and sexuality became the spoils of war of male deities. They became property to be used and controlled as the patriarchy saw fit. Time and again great spiritual beings emerge in the world and lead the people back toward a more egalitarian culture that worships the joy and pleasure of love and teaches respect for women. Jesus, who taught accountability and compassion, had female disciples who had equal status with their male counterparts, although I am doubtful you will find any fundamentalist Christians who will acknowledge the historical fact of female disciples. Nor did I ever hear at my Bible study group that women were at least coequal with men in receiving the Holy Spirit and prophetic gifts. After all, only women were present for the founding event of the church, Jesus's resurrection. They were also named apostles (Rom.16:7), disciples (Acts 9:36-42) and deacons (Luke 8:3) and led churches (Philem. 1-2). But this respect for women and recognition of their divinity was short-lived, as it always has been in the political history of all major religions.

Walter Wink, Professor of Biblical Interpretation at Auburn Theological Seminary, describes this period in Christianity's history in his profound book, *The Powers That Be:* "The tide, however, was turning. The vast majority of churches were soon dominated by male hierarchies, and women had been reduced to the roles of deaconesses and enrolled widows. Women who exercised authority were marginalized, accused of heresy, or silenced. Over time, men gained a monopoly on leadership in the church, and male supremacy demonstrated once more its resiliency under attack." Popular religious historian Karen Anderson said that the prophet Mohammed, the founder of Islam, had four wives who were enormously influential in the government after the prophet died. Throughout history, about a hundred years following the deaths of these various founders (Jesus, Mohammed, Buddha, Zoraster, Krishna), their religions have been taken over by patriarchal

Dominator forces. Religions were basically assimilated into the male power structure of the prevailing government. They take the heat of being a countercultural catalyst for a while, but then, in order not to share Jesus's punishment of torturous execution, they succumb to fear of torture and death, and sell out. This protects them from being viewed as a threat by the presiding patriarchal government. Then these religious leaders use the usual force and fear to collaborate with government leaders to maintain control over the people. They seldom speak out against their own governments, which provide them with protection. For example the Pope and the Catholic Church officially oppose the war in Iraq, but there has been almost no mention made of this in the media. Their moral compass gets lost when the state's enemies become the religion's enemies. Invariably these religious forces hoard power, accumulate wealth for the church, dominate and repress women and children, proclaim sexuality evil, and seek to be the controlling moral authority.

As a religion grows in numbers and gains power, Dominator governments also seduce and court the religious leaders by offering them special treatment and helping them in their missions. For example the same religious leaders of the Roman Empire that insisted on crucifying Jesus, and using Christians for lion chow, agreed to ban the practice of their "pagan" religion (which celebrated nature, sexuality and spirituality) within the Roman army. This removed what had been a major obstacle to Christians joining that army. Then they were able to join the same Roman Empire they had previously seen as evil, rationalizing that the army was necessary to protect the good Christian church from the evil of irreligious invading countries. But, as Wink writes,

> What killed Jesus was not irreligion, but religion itself; not lawlessness, but precisely the Law; not anarchy, but the upholders of order. It was not the bestial but those considered best, who crucified the one in whom divine Wisdom was visibly incarnate. And because he was not only innocent, but the very embodiment of true religion, true law, and true order,

this victim exposed their sacrificial violence for what it was: not the defense of society, but an attack against God.

Wink describes the mutual exploitation of the Roman Empire and Christianity:

> Christianity's weaponless victory over the Roman Empire resulted in the weaponless victory of the empire over the gospel. A fundamental transformation occurred when the church ceased being persecuted and became instead a persecutor. Once a religion attains sufficient power in a society that the state looks to it for support, that religion must also, of necessity, join in the repression of the state's enemies. For a faith that lived from its critique of domination and its vision of a nonviolent social order, this shift was catastrophic, for it could only mean embracing and rationalizing oppression.

Today, I heard on the British Broadcasting System that the governing body of those sweet, robe-wearing Buddhists was in an uproar because a woman had dared seek a position of authority within the religion in Thailand. Even though I wonder how this hijacking of compassion gets turned into control, I can already see the beginnings of it in our New Age spirituality movement. I was at a tantric puja gathering recently, ("puja" means prayer and "tantric" is about the bringing together of spirituality and physicality) and the facilitator told us to be careful that we did not indulge in any of that "lower chakra energy" (meaning sexual energy). He kept encouraging us to "elevate the energy" into the "higher chakras." Eisler makes the point this way: "I think one of the great tragedies of Western religion [and New Age spirituality] as most of us have known it has been its compartmentalized view of human experience, and particularly its elevation of disembodied or, 'spiritual' [higher chakra] love over embodied [lower chakra] or 'carnal' love."

One effect of this elevation of disembodied love is dissociation from that part of ourselves that feels empathy and compassion. Research shows that traditional religion, which supports the idea that God is out there beyond us, actually decreases our ability to feel compassion. Milton Rokeach, a professor at the University of Michigan, in his book *The Open and Closed Mind,* describes the research he did with groups of people from several of the world's major religions, including Christians and Jews. He gave them surveys which measured indices of compassion. He found that the more religious a person reported herself to be, the lower the scores she got for compassion. Rokeach also found that religious people generally scored less on compassion tests than non-religious people. The one exception he found was among the minorities within a religion. For example, religious blacks scored higher than whites.

You can not really tell whether an organization is serving life or not based on its cultural credibility, or its name, or even its stated intention. After the September 11th tragedy, quite a few compassioate-sounding organizations sprang up to "help the victims" but were later exposed as lining their own pockets. When an organization does have an invisible spiritual dimension to it, it is palpable. You can feel it when you walk in the door or attend the board meeting. Because I work with all kinds of organizations, churches, businesses and clubs, I get a lot of opportunities to notice, sense and feel their spiritual aspects. I have worked with certain churches that were reeking with fear, depression and hate—and others that uplifted my spirit just upon walking in the door.

One organization I've consulted for, John Paul Mitchell Systems (hair products and salons), has one of the sweetest, most spiritual vibrations of family I have ever experienced. This from a for-profit bunch of hair dressers—for God's sake! Every institution and each department has its own invisible spirit, atmosphere and culture. Every new venture, business, community or grass-roots organization starts with an intention. Author Walter Wink says each has its "angel" or spirit that determines its unique personality and what it brings into the world. Some of these spirits are more evolved and bring justice, non-violence, egalitarianism and abundance. Others manifest fear, greed, repression, control and domination.

If we intend to work with organizations, we will also need to address the root nature contained in their seed spirit. Some would say that it is just man's nature to want to be dominant. If that were true, then how could so many cultures have developed that are not based on dominance, but on cooperation? Ruth Benedict, in her book *Synergistic Societies,* writes about thirty-six such cultures.

The Choice of Natural Giving

I believe that humankind does not have a hard-wired nature of any kind, but it does have a choice about what values to live by. It's a choice to move towards partnership communities, where people are the partners of nature, women the equal partners of men, and whole communities the partners of children. Surely we could at least evolve to the level of certain species of monkeys like the Bonobos, whose society is not based on a hierarchical social system. Unlike the chimpanzee, the Bonobos do not have an alpha male that dominates the social order. Nor do they have violence to speak of, unlike the pugnacious chimps and most groups of human beings. Comparative psychologists suggest that this is due to the affectionate bonds that the female Bonobos make with each other, and the many cross-bonds between males and females. Chimps, on the other hand, use their male bonding to determine power relations, and to exert control over who gets how much food and when.

This does not happen with Bonobos. Because of the strong female bonding, males do not displace females at feeding sites, nor are they allowed to coerce sex from the younger or older females. Strong female bonding is a hallmark of nonviolent communities. Kuroda, a Kyoto University primatologist, suggests that another reason the Bonobos are "pacific, peaceful and gregarious" is because they have made an evolutionary movement toward sex as a means of creating a peaceful culture based on the sharing of sensual and sexual pleasure rather than on coercion and fear. All of the strong nonviolent matrilineal cultures that I have studied were based on the strength of the women's circle. At the Zegg Community the women meet together daily to clear the air between them and to strengthen, nurture and show affection for each other. This prevents divisive elements from growing and creates a powerful spiritual force field that will not tolerate any form of violence. It establishes a basis of trust between the women, one that prevents the fear and distrust that Dominator society women develop when it comes to their men. There is a trust and even an encouragement that the husbands of these women will be nurtured and loved by their sisters.

This kind of bonding is not allowed in totalitarian social systems like the fundamentalist Islamic Taliban societies. There are several common cultural norms that maintain a fundamentalist religious right's stranglehold of power over their people:

1. They keep the sexes separate in their schools and churches.

2. Sex is punished if used for anything other than procreation.

3. The head male in the family is religiously empowered to have exclusive control over women, children and sexual expression.

In Alice Miller's study of German family systems and culture, she describes how the tyrannical family unit, headed by a single strict dominating male, was one of the building blocks that allowed a Nazi government to do what it did. Wilhelm Reich, a refugee from Nazi Germany, said in his masterpiece *The Mass Psychology of Fascism* that historically, the best way for repressive governments to hold on to power was through the authoritarian family system, where its repressive ideology is indoctrinated into the next generation, particularly through what Reich calls "sexual suppression." He says the "psychosexual roots" of tyranny have a deep and long history.

It is a widespread dominator myth that if we have any intimacy or physical contact with someone, we must submit to sexual intercourse, go all the way. This myth is particularly sad for me. I have talked to a lot of people who do not know that they have permission to open up, have whatever degree of contact and intimacy they want—and then stop at whatever point they want. They do not know that they have no obligation to satisfy another's needs even if they did participate in a certain level of intimacy with that person. I wish everyone knew that they have permission to stop, guilt-free, and without having to explain or apologize. It is a tragedy that emotional intimacy, gentle touch, hand-holding, eye-gazing, skin-stroking, sensual warmth and emotional openness all often fail to occur because the culture of our communities does not affirm the sacred value and divine right of members to always be at choice.

In certain New Age communities that I have interacted with, hugging was not a choice, but an expectation. This turns a hug into a mug. These communities are covertly and unconsciously operating out of a patriarchal Dominator paradigm. An indication of this is that the idea of having a choice about the custom of hugging is not discussed. If someone does say "no" to a hug, there is often a reaction of hurt on the part of the person wanting to hug. They have a cultural judgement like, "You are just not a very open-hearted person like me." Most of the community members support this judgment, making it all the more difficult for people to stay at choice and in transparent truth.

I want communities to make it clear to their members that everyone has the right to stop the progression of any interaction at any time. The freedom to say "no" makes it safer to start saying "yes" to the sharing, affection and connectiveness that we are all so hungry for. In Dominator cultures, the word "no," when said by underlings, slaves, women or children, is punished.

One basis of this history comes out of our basic cultural building block: the traditional couple or marriage relationship. The norms and values for our Western marriage come from Europe, England and the Christian church. Eisler notes that

> The Church never took a vigorous position against the customary Germanic practice of men killing adulterous wives. Nor did it take a position against wife beating or the domination of women by men that it serves to maintain. In fact, the English common law governing marriage, which in large part is derived from earlier Church law, permitted a man to beat his wife if she did not perform her services to his satisfaction, just as slave owners were permitted to beat their slaves if they were not satisfied with them.

The Church also supported this sexual domination of women by men by making it a sin for the woman to ever say "no" to sex with her husband. Archbishop Stephen Langton suggested that the wife should allow herself to be killed before she allows her husband to go sexually unsatisfied, which might lead him to the great sin of adultery. So if a wife is to save her husband from the weeping and wailing of eternal hellfire, she must subjugate her own will to his and violate her own sacred sexuality.

Even the Free Love movement of the sixties was co-opted by the patriarchal paradigm that punishes women, for saying "no." They did this by making it "uncool" to say no to sex, and by the use of something perhaps even more painful than physical beating: shunning. Once you were labeled "uptight" and "unhip," you were no longer invited to be a part of that particular community's all-important party scene. "Free Love" came to mean giving up your free will to say, "No!" How ironic! Sometimes you can take the man out of the prison, but you can not take the prison out of the man.

The Dangers of Denying Our Sexual Natures

Because early church leaders were primarily celibate, which was — at least according to St. Paul — the highest spiritual path, they created a monastery culture of a lot of very frustrated (and therefore sexually obsessed) men.

It was from this breeding (or rather non-breeding) pool of men that the church chose the next leaders for their hierarchy. This created quite a constipation of testosterone in the church organization. And as with any part of ourselves that gets compartmentalized and cut off, it became obsessive/compulsive. This obsession got acted out, as most obsessions do, with a perverse need for control. The recent burst of scandals about Catholic priests molesting children shows what happens when the beast gets out of the closet. And the church, of course, has curled into a self-protective ball of denial.

In the case of the early church, this need for control got expressed by prying into the pajamas of both priests and parishioners. Priests' unconscious anger declared, "If we cannot enjoy any sex, then we are going to make sure you do not either!" Perhaps following St. Paul's often-quoted, "It is better to marry than to burn [in hell]," priests made any sex that is not solely for the purpose of procreating (and therefore never for love or pleasure) a damnable sin. It is strongly suggested in the Genesis story that the cause of the very fall of humankind was Eve tempting Adam with sex. This provides the Biblical basis for the broadly-held belief that women are simply to blame for everything.

I personally believe that Eve was framed by Domination-oriented Biblical editors. The effects of the combination of sexual repression — maintained through a delusion of spiritual superiority — and the power that Dominator organizations provide, are finally starting to be exposed. One or two sex scandals involving Catholic priests have turned into a nation-wide landslide of allegations. An institutional pattern has emerged, in which Bishops hid the abuses of priests. This reflects an institution wedded to denial.

I have worked with a number of people who have molested many children. Typically, they themselves were molested as children but learned to cope with the shame and humiliation by dissociating from their bodies and going up into their heads in daydreams of escape. In the same way, the hierarchy of the Church has dissociated from the body of the Church (the men, women and children who attend) in an attempt to protect the institution from damage. The system is seen as more sacred than the souls within it. This is another hallmark of a Domination organizational system. Although the priests who did the molesting and the bishops who cover it up are now being sacrificed on the altar of public opinion, the system that created and allowed these children to be used this way remains basically unquestioned.

I have seen many news stories about the life-long effects of abuse, and a few on what experts believe causes priests to stray. But most of the stories involve Protestant theologians talking about how wrong the cover up was and Catholic spin doctors defending child molestation as just a part of our society. One exceptional report presented a dramatic image of the Vatican's attitude. The story broke after the Pope called the American cardinals to Rome to talk about the priest child-molestation scandals in the U.S. One of the national networks, I believe ABC, reported that one of the Pope's closest cardinals had had many allegations of molestation leveled against him for many years— yet he was put in charge of a huge international residential program for young boys. An American reporter caught the Pope's liaison, who was identified as being the number-two-man in the Catholic Church, getting into his car. The reporter asked him what was being done about this cardinal. The cleric hit the reporter and refused to answer the question. He actually smacked him, just as though the reporter was his own abused child! What a perfect symbolic image: someone trying to get at the truth gets hit by the Powers That Be.

Certain family systems set the stage for children to be exploited. These family systems reflect the same principles and dynamics of the larger Domination hierarchy of which they are a part. Just as most traditional churches make sex a dirty subject not to be talked about, so it is within the family systems of so many of the victims. This is partly why it is taking so many years for the information about the abuse to come to light. (After the TV coverage of the molestations, a hotline was set up and is still deluged with new reports.) Another guiding darkness for these family systems is a Dominator interpretation of the fourth commandment: "Honor thy father and thy mother." This has been twisted to mean that no matter what your father and mother are doing to you, or telling you to do, you are to do it without question. This includes believing that Father O'Leary molested you, and Mother Superior hit you, for your own good, to help you transform your basically evil nature, which is there because you were born in original sin. To dishonor one's father or mother is to risk the wrath of a jealous male deity who sends little boys and girls into a fiery pit to be stabbed by pitchforks and tortured for eternity by a monstrous devil.

There is, by the way, no horned devil ever mentioned in the Bible. It was invented by the early Roman Christian church. It came from the image of the bull, with its horns, which was a symbol the Pagans and

Nature Worshipers held sacred as a symbol of abundance, potency, sexuality, and life. The church took their sacred symbol and used it to demonize the competing religion and justify the slaughter of around one million women herbalist-physician-priestesses who still worshiped the feminine aspect of the Goddess and nature in the third century. This literal demonization of their sacred symbol of sexuality, the bull, takes another interesting form. It appears in the slang expression "horny" as in "horny devil." Horny does not just mean sexually excited, lustful and aroused. In our sexually repressed culture it also means lascivious and lecherous. This association of sexual arousal with the Christian symbol of the incarnation of all that is carnal and evil, the devil, is no accident. If Christian leaders would acknowledge this mistake their religion has been making these last 1,700 years, it might begin to interrupt the dangerous dynamic of denial of this sacred part of ourselves. The consequences of religious repression of sex are deadly, although most major religions are in denial of this. This denial fits Scott Peck's definition of evil: "The central defect of evil is not the sin but the refusal to acknowledge it." I hope "60 Minutes" will one day report the effects that sexual repression and blind obedience to authority have on children and our society.

The Eroticization of Violence

This repressive control of the body and sexual behavior — particularly women's bodies and behavior — through the use of shame is the "ultimate mainstay of the Dominator social organization" according to Eisler. The early church amused itself by formulating thousands of rules dictating every aspect of sexual life. Even sexual positions were prescribed. Official doctrine on this point is found in the Codes Latinus Monacensis 22233. It tells us that the man must always be on top. Any departure from this is a sin as serious as murder. This position was divinely ordained because women were morally inferior and needed their evil natures to be controlled by men. All of this created what Eisler calls the "eroticization of dominance" in Western culture.

In American culture, this dominance is maintained by the eroticization of violence. Men's sexual arousal is addictively linked to a cycle of pursuit, seduction and eventual conquest of their prey, women. Just as Pavlov's dogs salivated when a bell was rung, Dominator cultures train men to associate the primary stimulus of a beautiful women's bodies with acts of violence and cruelty.

If you look at all the extremely violent video games that children are being trained by today: all the women being killed, as well as the heroines doing their share of maiming and slicing, you will notice that they are wearing very, very little clothing and have stereotypically huge breasts and exaggerated sexy bodies. In almost all the popular action movies, and most TV dramas, the hero kills the bad guy at the *climax* of the movie. Then he is rewarded by riding off into the sunset with a beautiful girl to have sex. After repeated associations, violence itself excites and arouses the man. This conditioning affects both men and women to the degree that cruelty and domination actually seem desirable and arousing to both sexes. There are many people who cannot even get sexually aroused without some sort of inflicted pain (whips) or domination (bondage).

In my clinical practice as a Marriage and Family Therapist I have worked with many marriages suffering from what traditional therapists label "disorder of desire." These couples have lost their erotic energy. One of the two, usually the woman, recognizes the unconscious demand for sex being placed on her by her husband. She rebels by resisting sex, which creates conflict. The more angry and hurt the man becomes in response to her need to assert her long-abandoned autonomy, the more the woman resists and avoids him.

Nonviolent Communication helps. As the man learns to have empathy for the emotional trauma his wife has suffered growing up in a woman-hating Dominator culture, he will give her the space to allow her sexual energy to emerge and blossom. If instead men continue to force themselves into women's psychosexual space, the quantity and quality of women's erotic energy will diminish. If men could have empathy for the woman's need for autonomy, respect and honoring, this would allow space for the great power of the feminine sexual nature to bloom in all it's vivacious glory. So it is really in men's interest to end the Dominator dynamic if they want more of that delicious loving, erotic, sensual, sexual energy in their lives.

When Violence=Pleasure

To change the Dominator dynamic within oneself, it is helpful to understand how it works. There are clinical experiments where men are shown five pornographic movies that have scenes linking sex and violence. The men are interviewed before and after viewing the films. Before watching the films the men were given tests to assess their attitudes toward male sexual violence toward women and whether they thought women enjoyed it. After watching the movies the men are much more likely to condone what the men in the movie did to the women and believe that the women enjoyed it. Also, instead of being disgusted by the violence, they were turned on by it, with pleasure hormones surging through their bodies.

This indicates that they were not only becoming desensitized to the violence, they were also beginning to develop an association between violence and pleasure. This creates a climate of fear for women. One fear is that if they do not obey men, they will be hurt. Another fear is that not only will men fail to protect them from other men who violate them, they will in fact be aroused by the violence. And it only takes a few acts of community-condoned violence to create such fear in the women that they dare not rock the boat. In my hometown of Brooksville, Florida, the Ku Klux Klan was respected for "keeping niggers in their place" — a code which meant keeping "our" women from violation by "them" blacks.

This use of violence to maintain control operates in family communities, too. I only had to get hit once by my physically abusive uncle to know that if I stepped out of line again I would get hit again. This social sanctioning of violence toward certain groups usually occurs in communities that teach the immorality of violence. The many Ku Klux Klansmen that I grew up with in Brooksville went to church every Sunday and would tell you that hurting people is wrong. But specific targeted violence was condoned as long as it "kept them niggers from getting too uppity" and kept the old boy's network in control.

It is particularly sad for me when I see members of such oppressed groups defending the very system that oppresses them. It is sad but also a predictable dynamic of oppressed people. I have worked for years with abused children who were removed from their homes. Invariably it is these same children who defend their parents' actions most vigorously. They cling to their parents out of their learned helplessness and dependency. This same dynamic keeps fundamentalist religious women defending traditional patriarchal marriage. Just as the slaves fought on the side of the south by the thousands to "preserve their way of life," women today sign up in droves for workshops to learn "The Rules" for tricking a man into a traditional marriage.

For those already married, there are books like *The Surrendered Wife*. Written by a woman, it teaches women to quit resisting the man's superiority. Maybe it should have been called *The Subjugated Wife*. I wish women particularly would quit joking that "if rape is inevitable you might as well learn how to enjoy it." I have also talked with African women who tell me that they support their own patriarchal cultural tradition of removing the clitoris of their daughters (again to prevent the women from being tempted to have sex outside of a possessive marriage). Over a hundred million African women have had their genitals mutilated in this way. The majority of them still support the practice as a sacred part of their cultural heritage. After all, they reason, it happened to them and they turned out to be good (meaning obedient) wives and mothers. I believe that this practice contributes to the loveless atmosphere in Africa that has led to so much war, cruelty and chaos. Whether in Afghanistan or Africa, the disempowerment of women comes before a great cultural tragedy. My heart still hurts when I remember the genocide in Rwanda. I doubt that the male tribal leaders of the Hutus and Tutsis could have lead their people to use machetes to hack to death close to a million people if their women had been culturally empowered, rather than subjugated.

Some would say that no one has a right to interfere with another's culture. I suggest these people smoked too much pot and watched too much Star Trek in the 'sixties. Remember the prime directive of Star Fleet? It was "To never interfere with the development of another civilization." Such noble philosophy can disconnect us from our hearts and rationalize apathy. I imagine after a couple of hundred years, the "cultural tradition" of sending Jews to the gas chambers would have become part of the consecrated culture of the Nazis, had they survived.

When a man is highly sexually aroused but dissociated from his emotions, he is able to do things to women that he could not otherwise do. Without dissociation he might feel empathy for the women's pain and fear. His conscience might stop him. This is important to understand because this is also how boys are socialized to be violent. Boys are trained to feel a sexy powerful surge of good feelings whenever they are dominating someone. They are trained to identify with the aggressor and disidentify with the weak, disgusting victim. After all, who do you want to be: Superman or the cowardly weasel he is crushing? In Dominator cultures, the military trains testosterone-charged young men to suppress their natural empathy and kill and hurt people. I do not think it is necessary for a country to use this tactic to create a strong army. But American army culture still engages in the domination of women, as we saw in the Tailhook scandal. Women were sexually assaulted in order to keep them "in their place" and prevent them from attaining the rank of pilot.

I found this same contempt for the feminine, and for soft or caring sex, among military men and teachers in Belgrade, Serbia. This is the same military that, under orders from their government, raped tens of thousands women and children in Bosnia. During the Bosnian war, when I was asked by the Psychology Department of the University of Belgrade to teach their psychologists how to help the victims to heal, I discovered that of the 60 psychologists in the group only one was male. In Montenegro, where many raped refugees fled to get away from the Serbian army, I also found that almost the entire group of therapists was female. Their case loads sometimes numbered in the hundreds.

The male university teachers typically scoffed at me when I taught Nonviolent Communication classes. Their culture had taught them fear of feelings, releasing control, soft sexuality and the feminine—a fear typical of Dominator systems. Men are taught that to have empathy or care for anyone outside their group will result in their being exploited and victimized. Little boys are socialized from the beginning to see the feelings useful for dominating people (anger and contempt) as masculine. Sadness, fear and compassion are seen as feminine. The masculine feelings are portrayed as superior, and the feminine feelings are portrayed as inferior and associated with weakness. Little boys are taught: "Don't cry. Get mad, then get even." This hatred for the soft and the feminine is also a hatred for love, life, sexuality and indeed caring of any kind.

It is ancient tradition that the spoils of war include raping the women of your conquered foe. At the close of World War II the Russian army is said to have raped every woman in Berlin between eight and eighty. Young suicide bomber martyrs are promised fifty virgins in heaven if they do their deadly duty to their God and their people. The Christian church's equation of sex with sin, damnation and guilt creates a great fear of true intimacy between men and women. It puts men in their heads, hypervigilant about what the "right" thing to think or do is, dissociated from the bodies in which those painful emotions and evil impulses reside. Now who determines what the "right" thing to think and do is? Why the church, of course!

It is this dissociation from the body, with its emotions of empathy, compassion and caring, that makes it possible for people to participate in the painful domination of others and even to allow themselves to be made into slaves. What prevents rebellion from breaking out? Alice Miller says it is the use of the concept that all the control and punishment is done "for your own good." This is also the title of one of her many excellent books. In other words, you are being dominated to protect you from going to Hell. You fit into your Dominator society so you will not be punished, starved or shunned. If the church can convince you that pleasure is bad and pain is good, then maybe it is not bad to cause pain to others, as long as you do it for their own good.

Without this kind of dissociation from the body and abandonment of one's own inner compassionate empathic authority, we never would have had the Church's Inquisitions, Crusades, religious schools, corporal punishment, and witch-burnings.

From Coercive to Compassionate Community

If something has gotten in the way of our natural joy in giving to each other, let us sit together and uncover it again. That joy is our interconnectedness, our amoebic oneness of organism. It can never be destroyed, only buried beneath the hurts of our misperception of each other's intentions. It is very easy for this interconnectedness to get lost in the push-pull polarization of the basic relational unit of society, the couple unit. It may be that the human being is a tribal or pack animal, like wolves and giraffes, and not like swans that travel and live in pairs. The strength and security that a tribe supplies is essential to preventing the usual codependency in couple relationships. Without this strength of emotional and spiritual security, clinging is inevitable, which is poison to love. Here is how Paul Ferrini in his book *Love Without Conditions* describes this dynamic: "Compassion and detachment go hand in hand. You cannot love someone and seek to control him. Only by wanting what is best for him do you offer your brother freedom. And if you do not offer him freedom, you do not offer him love."

Every situation in your life provides you with an opportunity to gain greater intimacy and greater freedom. As you love more and more people more and more deeply, you become less attached to them individually. You become attached not to the specific person, but to the love that each one extends to you. This is a movement toward the experience of Divine Love which is beyond the body, indeed beyond form of any kind.

Many "primitive" cultures cannot understand our "advanced" Western civilization. They cannot understand how we could abandon a mother to raise her child basically by herself. They do not know how we can stand the isolation of our little cookie-cutter neighborhoods. They are saddened by our lack of purpose and service and expression in daily life. Here is a reaction, from tribal leader Sobonfu Somé from the African Dagara tribe, to how we in the West try to make the couple substitute for community. This is from her book *The Spirit of Intimacy: Ancient African Teachings:*

It's very strange to regard two people as a community. Where is everybody else? Community is the spirit, the guiding light of the tribe, whereby people come together in order to fulfill a specific purpose, to help others fulfill their purpose, and to take care of one another. The goal of the community is to make sure that each member of the community is heard and is properly giving the gifts he has brought to this world. Without this giving, the community dies.

There seems to be an interdependent ecology needed for peaceful communities to occur. It starts with an individual feeling the significance, belonging, freedom to love as she sees fit, and the security of knowing her niche in the fabric of her community. Without this security, an unconscious collective insecurity develops in the culture. It manifests itself in the forms of pillaging nature, war between the sexes, and fraternal cultures like the Israelis and Palestinians attacking each other. When this security is restored, a flow of loving relationing can occur at every level.

What is the genesis of our cultural insecurity?

Dieter Duhm of the Zegg community has founded "healing biotopes" to counter cultural insecurity. A biotope is a consciously created environment, based on ecological principles that support a partnership social organization, for nurturing the creative expression and rapid evolution of human beings. Duhm talks about the foundation of our cultural insecurity:

The Judeo-Christian culture has two key principles that form the spiritual backbone of its cultural paradigm. One is the idea of a punishing god which keeps the majority of the culture under a blanket of controlling fear. The second is the ancient myth of love and the belief that love and jealousy are inseparable. This idea is not only false, it is self-contradictory.

Jealousy is not a part of love; it is an obstacle to love. It is the death of love. As long as the traditional sacrament of marriage remains so closely linked to possessiveness, jealousy will continue to rant and rage. No violence-free Earth, no sexpeace and no permanent love will be allowed to develop, neither on an individual basis between lovers nor as a catalyst for an overall culture. In ecological, military, and human terms, nothing has devastated our Earth more than the fatal guiding mechanism of this false conception of love. Nothing else has been more to blame for driving us to loneliness, despair, grief and cynicism. And nothing else has produced so many mental and physical diseases as the eternal waiting for fulfillment which is impossible under these circumstances. This should be included in the diagnosis of almost every psychosomatic illness: patient is suffering from an incurable lovesickness caused by a false conception of love.

This false conception of love is maintained through the institution of patriarchal traditional marriage. Traditional "Holy Matrimony" is really an unholy and wholly unfair business transaction and has the same pathetic dynamics as the institution of prostitution. Riane Eisler makes the same point:

> The assumptions behind prostitution as an economic transaction through which men purchase women's bodies are actually not so very different from the contractual assumption behind "traditional marriage." For the traditional marriage contract (like the agreement between a man and a prostitute) is essentially also one of power imbalances: one through which the less powerful woman unconditionally sells her body to the more powerful man. Hence the failure even to this day, in some American states, to recognize marital rape as a crime rather than a "natural" aspect of a husband's entitlement to his wife's sexual services in conformance to stereotypical masculine and feminine gender roles.

This false conception of love is also supported by how some of the writings in our great religions anthropomorphize God. Many ancient writers projected their own human weakness onto their image of God, thereby not only releasing themselves of guilt, but making the quality of jealousy holy and blessed. The desire for the jealous control over others becomes a good, noble and righteous quality. In the Old Testament we read that God is a jealous God and will not tolerate any other God (sounds a little insecure to me). There are similar passages in Islam, Hinduism, and other world religions. These provided the intellectual justification for Crusades, Inquisitions, jihads and other holy wars, not to mention certain acts of terrorism involving tall buildings. The idea that the Gods of these different religions are jealous contributes to the justification for conquering someone else's society.

It also sanctifies religious patriarchies in the hallowed practice of the domination of women, children and sexuality. Of course this domination is said to be done only "for their own good," presumably to protect them from their inherently evil, selfish and sexual nature. The founding fathers of Christianity debated as to whether a woman even had a soul. It is ironic that although women are seen as worth less in fundamentally religious cultures, the degree of the male's possessiveness of her is much greater here than in other cultures. There have been many news stories lately of the "honor" killings of women in fundamentalist Muslim countries like Saudi Arabia. In Afghanistan under the Taliban, wives, sisters and daughters could be legally stoned to death if they are suspected of fraternizing with an unapproved male. They may also be killed if they have been seen or touched or raped against their will. They are killed by their fathers, brothers and husbands, not to punish the women but to simply dispose of damaged property. The woman is thought to have brought shame on the man or family, not through an immoral act or fault in character, but because she is no longer a virgin or has been sullied and therefore her value as an object has been lost. By killing her, the family "honor" has been restored. Schmookler writes that "sexual possessiveness is the pulsating heart of honor."

This kind of possessiveness is not limited to fundamentalist Muslim countries, as I have discovered in my marriage counseling practice with thousands of couples. The primary paradigm for "Love American Style" is one based on mutual possessiveness. Cultural anthropologist James Prescott discovered that this possessiveness occurs much more often in societies that emphasize military glory and worship aggressive gods. Schmookler agrees that "there does seem to be a connection between the high valuation of sexual fidelity (the granting, particularly by the woman, of exclusive sexual possession) and cultural bellicosity." Schmookler later suggests that the sense of scarcity and possessiveness that drives men to war also kills the flow of love between men and women. He thinks that it is "less moral evil than spiritual ignorance." He calls this ignorance "a fundamental mis-apprehension of the way life is" and a "misguided approach to rela-tionship because it comes from a spiritual condition antagonistic to true fulfillment."

True fulfillment must follow the flow of life. This flow requires that we not try to possess or hoard life, but allow air to come into and out of our lungs, and food to enter and leave our bodies. Schmookler writes about how the basic unit of society, the man/woman relation-ship, is corrupted by man's false pride and lack of faith: "The man of honor's possession of his cherished female reveals a kind of Midas touch: the possibilities of genuine relationship are forfeited, killed by the transmutation of a living human being into a mere object. An image of this is found in the grotesque chastity belts employed by the medieval man of war to safeguard his treasure of flesh and blood dur-ing his absence."

Riane Eisler says that the distortion of sexuality — the equating of masculinity with both sexual and social domination, and equating femininity with sexual and social submission — is critical to the main-tenance of a Dominator social organization. This distortion of sexuali-ty into an issue of honor and a "pride of possession" is central particularly to the male's socialization into domination and violence. It is this same false conception of love that is the meat and potatoes of Pop Psychology in America. Quoting again from the June 2000

Psychology Today article, "Jealousy — Why we need it as much as love and sex," the writer proclaims, "If he reacts to her flirtations with emotional indifference, she knows he lacks commitment; if he gets jealous, she knows he's in love." (page 60) Wow! There it is in black and red, white and blue. I can see a new dot com company forming now:, "Girls! Tired of the same old commitment-phobic men? Get online now and get hooked up with a man who will never leave and knows how to commit. Just log on at www.Stalkers.com.

Jealousy is a part of love in the same way that asthma is a part of breathing. Nor are fear and shame a part of spirituality. I think that in order to have a true conception of love, we need to develop unconditional trust in our relationships and personal potency within ourselves. Without unconditional trust we cannot have unconditional love. By unconditional trust I mean a trust without a "that" behind it. So unconditional trust would not say, "I trust *that* you will always take care of me" or, "that you will always feel affectionate or sexual towards me" or, "that you will always remember my birthday" or, "that you will love only me." True trust or faith, as in faithfulness, sets no conditions or expectations: "I trust you to follow you soul's agenda for love and growth and I trust myself to do the same. As we support each other in this process, our trust in each other grows.

It is very difficult to hold this consciousness of unconditional trust outside a collective field of energy, one that gets created by a community of people holding a certain consciousness and intention. This group of connected potent people must value unconditional trust and transparency.

Without this energy field of unconditional trust, there will always be a hiding of shameful and guilty feelings, thoughts and actions. Hiding these things gives people an explosive, compulsive power that often leads to physical illness or uncontrollable destructive action. These actions include things like the secret affairs that America seems so addicted to and fascinated by. One of the most popular TV shows in our culture is Jerry Springer, which is forever feeding our fascination with covert sexuality. I know people who almost lost their jobs because they got sucked into the vortex of mass hysteria by compulsively watching the Bill and Monica media.

The group mass mind is not only addictive, it is contagious, for better or for worse. And the group mass mind is a terrible thing to waste. James Redfield, author of *The Celestine Prophecy*, wrote about the nature of this shared mind and its potential for creating a loving culture in his spiritual thriller *The Secret of Shambhala:*

> "...What you are understanding is the contagious aspect of the human mind," Yin explained. "In a sense, we all share minds. Certainly we have control over ourselves and can pull back, cut ourselves off, think independently. But as I said earlier, the prevailing human worldview is always a giant field of belief and expectation. The key to human progress is to have enough people who can beam a higher expectation of love into this human field. This effort allows us to build an ever higher level of energy, and to inspire each other toward our greatest potential...."

Apathy, Community and Consumerism

Our consumer complex may threaten civilization more than the military industrial complex. We must earn more and more money to create wider and wider wide-screen TVs with more and more picture resolution and higher quality surround sound with more channels. One of the purposes of this great marketing machine is to get us to confuse strategies and needs. It spends billions to figure out how to convince us that we "need" a Big Mac or a Toyota Camry. In reality we need food and transportation. Big Macs and Camrys are strategies, i.e. one specific way, among many possibilities, for meeting the basic, underlying need. The potency of our culture is being siphoned off to support and defend this complex. The hunger to consume and consume is like salt water: the more you drink the more you thirst. The more we watch TV, the emptier we feel—so we watch more TV.

Just as Bill W. discovered that the solution to his drinking problem was his AA community, our consumerism-trying-to-fill-our-emptiness-problem is solved by a certain quality of encounter with community. If we don't find or create this community for ourselves, we unwittingly continue to support the Great American Consumer Complex. The new community must have the high voltage electricity of connection flowing through it to compete with the electronic entertainment that the Consumer Complex is offering. This will require us to rethink our attitudes about love, sexuality, intellectualism and spirituality. If we pull away from the toys and toward each other, we experience an enormous flow of power, love and creativity. We experience potency, worthiness, validation and connectedness with other individuals, our community and Mother Earth.

When I give my energy to another and see how it brings the light back to their eyes, I know I am of tremendous value. When another gives me their uncensored attention and I feel the rush of life energy on every level pulsate through me, I truly know in that moment that life is very, very good. My connection and trust for this grows, and a basis for working and playing together grows. Then we can truly start to form conscious compassionate creative "community".

I asked Hans de Boor, the famous German statesman, author, and student of Gandhi: "Gandhi said that for every thousand who are chopping at the leaves of the tree of violence, only one is chopping at the root. What is the root, in your opinion?" He replied: "Apathy is the new Fascism and Nazism. We all know what is happening on this planet, just as I, as a member of Hitler's Youth, knew what my government was doing. We could smell the burning of human flesh coming from the so-called 'factories,' but we busied our minds with other things."

So we must first end the apathy, oppression and depression in our own communities. This oppression comes from religious and social traditions that make sexuality and spirituality a patented religious franchise and potency the property only of those presently in authority. Our opulent culture is still using consumerism and addictions to dull the pain caused by the loss of the original love of life, the world of nature and family. The New Community is not a utopian dream but a chance for a glorious, mysterious, passionate adventure into a fully lived life.

Our being painfully nice has made us depressed, but it has also deprived the world of our passion for making it a better place for all of humankind. If we could throw off the oppression of our own niceness, we would be able to recover our innate passion for creating a new just and compassionate culture.

Chapter

CREATING THE NEW CULTURE

The journey toward a more conscious culture begins by cultivating an attitude of true tolerance and holistic forgiveness. Those holding an attitude of unconditional trust do not interpret inevitable human violations as a breech of trust. When a community supports interpretations of this kind, it serves to tear at the fabric of all relationships and can be totally destructive to the family structure. I wish some of Washington, D.C.'s fundamentalist "Family Values" lobbyists could work with me for a day as a Family Therapist and see the effect their "ethics" have on families. Once they have a whole community supporting them in their religious rage about someone having "cheated" or "lied" or been "permissive" with their children, it is hard to get them to come down out of their judgmental heads and practice what Jesus taught: forgiveness and understanding, compassion, empathy, respect, egalitarianism and unconditional love. Just as the Roman Empire began to wage war against the early Christians, throwing them in lion pits and crucifying them, today's fundamentalist establishment has declared war "for the soul of the nation." Their banner reads, "Return to Family Values." Eisler writes that this term is a code word for "an authoritarian, male-dominated, patriarchal family designed to teach both boys and girls to obey orders from above [be nice], no matter how unjust or unloving they may be."

The leaders of this campaign are the wealthy WASP male heads of fundamentalist and other religious groups who interpret their holy books to read that men should rule over women and nature. They believe that the cause of our social problems is a lack of male control over women, children and sexuality. I believe that this dominating control, and ranking of men over women and children, is a great cause of the lack of love in our society. These leaders would return to the system that Jesus tried to change, a millennia-old Roman Empire system of rule by the hierarchical male heads of households.

Counter Your Culture's Norms

I would suggest we adopt Jesus's family values, where Joseph never once dominated or punished Mary or Jesus (even when he ran off without permission and was studying in the temple), but treated them as his divine equals. Throughout the New Testament in every encounter Jesus has with women, he violates the prevailing customs in ways that demonstrate caring and respect for the women and disregard for the discriminative laws of his "civilization." It was considered immoral at the time for men and women to be traveling around together, as Jesus and his male followers did with Mary Magdalene and Joanna, who provided financially for the disciples. He was truly chopping at the *root* of violence, which is the elevation of one part of humanity over another.

Whether it is the caste system of India, the apartheid of Africa or our own beloved forms of patriarchy, there is a common element. Walter Wink writes,

> No matter how high in the patriarchal social order a woman might rise, she was always controlled by men sexually and reproductively. Every class had two tiers, one for men, and a lower one (in the same class) for women. Power lost by men through submission to a ruling elite was compensated for

by power gained over women, children, hired workers, slaves and the land. In the increased violence and brutality of the new order, it was in the interest of women to seek out a male protector and economic supporter. But the price they paid was sexual servitude, undervalued domestic labor, and subordination to their husbands in all matters. As a fringe benefit, women were permitted to exploit men and women in races or classes lower than their own. Those in power created or evolved new myths to socialize women, the poor, and captives into their now-inferior status. Priesthoods, back up by armies, courts of law and executioners, inculcated in people's minds the fear of terrible, remote and inscrutable deities. Wife-beating and child-beating began to be seen as not only normal but a male right. Evil was blamed on women.

This dominator system is our heritage. I'll give a personal example of how our religions support and promote this system of inequality: when I was a child, our community centered around a certain Baptist Church. Our family of six had run into difficult financial times, so my father humbled himself and asked the church if they could help us with some groceries. The only response from the minister was a Bible verse: "The poor will always be with you." When my father was put in prison for stealing to feed his four children, the church condemned him for it. After a few years of my father's imprisonment, my mother had an affair, and the church condemned her for it. When my father got out of prison he left my mother, driven by the shame and shunning our church offered him. It was not long before the social workers came and sent us off into different foster homes. Our family was never reunited. This is the fate of too many families in America. This morality of conditional love and condemnation is tearing families apart.

An alternative is the practice of unconditional love and trust. These values remind me to look for the always understandable (but not necessarily condonable) reasons for each other's behavior. These reasons are often mixed with misunderstandings, false beliefs and past pain. Unconditional trust keeps me conscious of the inevitable healing, and reconnection in love for each other, that occurs if we continue to practice empathy for each other. This effort to keep having empathy for each other must be supported by a closely knit community. The fact that our culture does not know how to support couples and families emotionally is a primary cause of the disintegration of families. Mental health philosophers have recognized that a child acting out in an alcoholic family is labeled the "identified patient," recognizing the child as part of a dysfunctional family system. But we still think of a couple having problems as being a dysfunctional couple. Maybe they are just the "identified patient" within a dysfunctional community system. Part of the problem with our thinking is that we often consider couples to be a complete little system, closed unto itself.

The Closed Circle of Incest

The reasons for this go way back in history. Margaret Mead, the great anthropologist, said that we developed the closed nuclear family some hundreds of years ago as a response to the many wars that were occurring. Small nuclear families were much more mobile and could not only flee war more effectively but also start over in a new location more easily. Mead says we lived in tribes or clans of between twelve and thirty-six people for many thousands of years before the nuclear family arose.

Another big historical reason for keeping a tightly closed couple system is to protect men's property rights. What property am I referring to? His wife and children. Have you ever heard the term "rule of thumb?" It comes from an early British law that said that you were not allowed to beat your wife with a stick larger than your thumb—in your legal attempt to make her keep the "obey" part of the "love-honor-and-obey" marriage vow.

If you want to understand the effects and dynamics of a closed social system, study incestuous families. Everything is controlled by one person in the family in order to prevent the "dirty laundry" from being aired. The metaphorical drapes of the house are drawn. Little in-depth interaction with other people is allowed, which prevents any understanding of what healthy interaction feels like. In this closet system, self-worth plummets, while fear of abandonment and a desperate sense of dependency keep shameful secrets secret.

Closed social systems are like little stagnant ponds that breed all the vile reptiles of the human psyche. Open social systems are like rushing rivers that give fresh life and perspective to the soul.

In the book *Hot and Cool Sex*, Anna and Robert Francoeur quote Professor Ray Birdwhistell, a family psychiatrist who studied the expectations of the model American family, which he traces back to the late nineteenth century:

> This model contained two main components: the first, the "fantastic" notion that one man and one woman should be responsible for satisfying all of each other's emotional needs; the second, the idea that parents should be responsible for meeting all their children's needs. Birdwhistell uses terms like "cannibalistic," "exotic and impossible," to describe these two expectations, and rightly so. The ideal is never achieved in life, yet it is a very real social model that turns the home into a cage. "Caging," Birdwhistell suggests, is accomplished by reducing meaningful lateral contacts, especially for the parents. Parents and children exist in a self-enclosed unit. Relationships outside the cage are formal and impersonal, and contribute little, if anything, to personal growth and development. Children are raised in this emotional cage and, when old enough, pushed out to set up their own cages, from the isolated cages of suburban homes and urban condominiums and tenements to the smaller cages of reservations reserved for the aged, our "leisure villages."

Couples Need Caring Communities

The whole question of nonviolent societies, peace on earth, dominance and submission, oppressor and oppressed, and even Rodney King's, "Can't we just get along," is reflected within the dysfunctional couple dynamic. Any culture's generalized couple dynamic is a hologram or symbolic representation of the whole culture. You can understand what's wrong with a culture by understanding what's wrong with its couples. Virginia Satir used to portray the American Couple through the use of body sculpting. First she would portray the male by standing with an angry, contemptuous expression, pointing a shaming index finger downward toward a groveling, cowering, sniveling, crying woman, curled up on the floor with folded hands, apologetically begging for mercy. In any system: family, culture or organization, if you can convince people that it is a part of love to withhold love or to punish another for their own good, you can create a master/slave culture.

Punishment and the withholding of love must be replaced by the skillful use of presence, by egalitarian negotiation using honest and empathetic dialog, and by the protective use of force based on self-compassion. This use of force must never by used to punish but only to insure that needs that are nonnegotiable get met. In my family I use this force to stop my two-year-old from running into the street. I use as little force as is necessary to meet my own need to have her be safe. I use this force only until I can educate her about necessary street precautions and convince her of my value for safety.

In a community, a person doing harm to others must be isolated until they can receive the empathy they require in order to be empathic to others. The empathy they would then be able to feel for others would prevent them from doing harm to others. They would be educated in alternative ways of getting their needs met, ones that are not at someone else's expense.

In the Zegg community, as in many intentional communities, it is understood that when two people are not getting along, it affects the whole community's emotional atmosphere. The ecological interdependence of the basic unit of relationship, the couple, and the larger unit of the community is recognized and consciously addressed. This is vastly different than what happens in most American subcultures, where a couple's problems are seen as their own private business.

There is also an understanding that problems cannot be solved on at the same level as they were created. When couples at the Zegg community have problems, the problems are taken on as a community project. The community supports each individual to withdraw the polarizing projection and take responsibility for asserting whatever their needs are within the community. Dieter Duhm says, "Jealousy especially cannot be worked out by the couple alone. An inner group coherence based on transparent structures can grow and develop only if the pair can open themselves and trust the group with their internal difficulties. Without this trust the couple stays in their closed system and usually develops some dysfunctional adaptation to it. They go dead in their relationship, move to separate parts of the house or enter a superficial fantasy relationship."

Jealousy is a form of attachment and can also be a type of addiction. Coercing your husband or girlfriend to listen to you for extended periods of time about your pain of jealousy may contribute to your own fear that you cannot feel okay without that particular person's attention. It may be useful to go to other people and certainly to your journal to get the empathy and mirroring you need to reestablish connection with your faith, confidence, potency, and inner security.

When I go to my beloved for empathy about the jealousy I feel, it is like going to my heroin pusher for drug addiction counseling. Anything I get from her will increase my dependence on her. The fact that I am jealous indicates that I am overly dependent on her. I am only jealous toward people I am trying to get my self-worth from. This jealousy arises from a belief that having her exclusive attention creates my feelings of self-worth. Believing that my self-worth lies outside of my own control leaves me feeling painfully powerless and triggers a compulsive need to control my beloved. It is this compulsion to control that kills. In his book *The Heart of Man*, Erich Fromm characterizes this dynamic as similar to that of the necrophile (one who loves the dead). Fromm says the necrophile "can relate to an object—a flower or a person—only if he possesses it." Such possessiveness is not love at all, but rather a compulsive need to control. "In the fact of controlling," Fromm says, the person "kills life."

This need to control, which is a central dynamic in jealousy, comes from an unconscious sense of powerlessness. Rollo May writes: "Jealousy characterizes the relationship in which one seeks more power than love. It occurs when the person has not been able to build up enough self-esteem, enough sense of his own power, his own 'right to live.'" As people mature they are better able to become deeply involved and committed in a spiritual, sexual partnership without possessiveness and jealousy. When someone supports her partner's jealousy, by making costly, unwanted behavior changes or processing her partner's pain longer than she wants to, it is often because of a sense of guilt about her actions, or her own fear of loss of connection with her mate. Over time this leads to resentment. Her allegiance is given from fear and guilt, and not from the heart. When jealousy is supported as a value in a community, everyone hates everyone else who has power or attractiveness. This also makes it difficult for anyone to let his light shine, because to do so runs the risk of being shunned by the majority of his sex.

This general insecurity in the community makes it difficult for anyone to own his power. The men hate other powerful men for the shame they feel when comparing themselves to them. They also fear them for different reasons, including that they may take their women away. Some women hate and fear women who have potency, because they, too, compare themselves unfavorably and fear they will lose their men to them. These dynamics of jealousy and possessiveness contribute to creating thousands and thousands of social circles all across the country based on fear, competition and an unreasonable sense of scarcity. The shallowness of these circles leave their members empty, looking for Mr. Right (or even Mr. Right Now!) to fill the hole in the their souls.

Virginia Satir said, "There are no bad people, only bad rules that create bad systems." These bad systems do two things. First, they confuse the truth with its opposite, by suggesting that things like fear of loss and jealousy are love. Secondly, they advocate the value of cutting off and repressing parts of human nature, particularly our power, our bodily emotions and the fullness of our sexual nature. Many sociologists and psychologists are now coming into agreement about the link between repressed instincts and drives to cruelty. And many doctors are now documenting the connection between this repression and illness. Here are some suggestions to help you tame the Green-eyed Monster:

First Aid After the Jealousy Button's Pushed

1. Call a time out and see if you can get your emotions and imagination back under your control.

2. Set a time limit about how long you will try to deal with it on your own.

3. Reach out for support if you exceed your time limit.

4. Journal down all the dynamics, your thoughts and feelings and needs, to read to your support group.

5. Re-Source. Your jealousy has just made someone else your source, and you have lost connection with your true inner source.

6. Instead of asking your self "why is this happening to me?" Start asking your higher power/self/source "what am I to learn from this situation?"

Preventive Medicine for Jealousy

1. Put energy into your own passions and purposes. If you are not clear on what they are, ask yourself the questions Jean Houston suggests: "What do you ache for? ...Are you willing to risk looking like a fool for love, your dreams and the adventure of being alive?" (If this frightens you and stimulates images of being a bag lady living under a bridge, read *Do What you Love and the Money will Follow*, by Marsha Sinetar.) When people have a passion and a purpose, they do not make their partner the sole source of their self-worth. This protects them from the compulsion to control this sole source.

2. Seek a passionate spirituality.

3. Become involved in the creation of a non-judgmental transparent community.

4. Receive strong doses of yin and yang energy. Create a same-sex support group and really steep yourself in the nurturing that only your own sex can give you. This will create such a concentration and polarization of either female/yin or male/yang energy that you will become very attractive to the opposite sex in a potent, powerful and passionate way. Then indulge yourself in the rich, sexy, creative, loving reunion of pure opposites.

5. Make a clear contribution to your community and receive recognition for it.

Catalyzing Cultural Change Within

So where to start creating this cultural change that is so desperately needed? Gandhi said we must be the change we seek to see in the world. Dieter Duhm said it this way:

What then follows is cultural work with ourselves and the way we lead our daily lives. Our suffering is a signal from a life that is not lived. Healing consists of recognizing—and living—that "unlived" life. To surmount our deeply engrained restraints, our fears and weariness, our much too cozy humanness, and our alternative gardens of refuge, we need an experimental milieu in which such a transformation is understood and affirmed. We need an inner centering and free communication outwards. That is the key for a new culture. It includes new forms of living together, raising children, new forms of love and sexuality. The creation of a life-oriented culture requires the creation of a new social and emotional space where people can again learn to live and breathe freely. Such places would create the most dependable healing power against fear and hatred—love.

Many new leaders in the quest for this life-oriented culture are emerging and pointing the way to a more enlightened ethics, as Eisler describes here:

Some writers, such as the anthropologist Gayle Rubin, have taken the position that a new sexual ethic should revolve primarily around whether sex is consensual. However, she qualifies this by adding that—rather than the traditional division between acceptable or good sex as heterosexual, married, monogamous, and reproductive, and bad sex as anything else—sexual acts should be judged, "by the way partners treat one another, the level of mutual consideration, the presence or absence of coercion, and the quantity and quality of the pleasure they provide." This new culture would have as the measure of morality the value of consensus instead of conformity or coercion. It would stress compassion, instead of control, pleasure instead of pain. This would apply to all areas of human interactions, whether it be sexuality, business, government, family life or communication. But because sexuality is the spiritual core of our love and physical life, and the linchpin that Dominator forces use to accumulate power over societies, these new ethics must apply most vigorously to our sexuality.

Eisler describes the process of developing the new culture as a shift in paradigms. She writes,

> If we succeed in completing the cultural shift from a dominator to a partnership social and ideological organization, we will see a real sexual revolution—one in which sex will no longer be associated with domination and submission but with the full expression of our powerful human yearning for connection and for erotic pleasure. It will be a sexuality that will make it possible for us to more fully express and experience sexual passion as an altered state of consciousness. It will also bring the recognition that erotic pleasure can be imbued with a spirituality that is both immanent and transcendent. And it will combine greater sexual freedom with greater empathy, respect, responsibility, and caring.

This new culture would not value being one of the nice, dead, conforming "sheeple" of the community, but would value holistic selfishness based on an awareness of the unity of life. It would value service to the collective society, but not at the expense of the individual and honor the ecological interrelationship between ourselves, nature and each other.

The ability to control how love and sexuality are dispensed allows the dynamic of domination to emerge in a couple or in a culture. Love and sexuality can be spiritual forces for the nurturing of harmony within individuals and groups as long as the sacredness and primacy of free will and autonomy is maintained.

As we begin to practice this new partnership paradigm of relating and organizing, we will necessarily meet a great deal of resistance from the status quo. We will encounter it within ourselves as the fear of change, within our families as an attempt to maintain homeostasis, and within our social structures as the fear of loss of the current political and economic power structures. A prominent Jewish friend of mine was participating in local Jewish-Arab dialogues in San Diego. In the course of these dialogues she stated her position against the use of violence of any kind whether it be Arab or Israeli. Since then, she has been receiving enormous amounts of criticism from a number of local Jews, including some threats. So we need to be prepared for many of our loved ones and people in our present community to judge us as odd, immoral, left wing, radical, sissy, pathological, idealistic, disloyal and wrong.

> -§-
> You cannot contribute to one person in a relationship. What ever you do, it serves both or neither.
> -§

Violence Is a Boomerang!

Violence will never work because even when it works, it fails. As Wink points out "violence can never stop violence because its very success leads others to imitate it. Ironically, violence is most dangerous when it succeeds."

Our challenge will be to resist our reptilian brain's inclination to perceive attack, triggering an unconscious flight-or-fight response. We can begin to develop an alignment with the principles of nature and an enlightened form of self-interested morality, if we can truly make the connection between what we put out and what comes back at us. When we express the energy of judgment, domination, coercion, hate and violence outwardly, we will most likely trigger the same response from others. This is true whether we do it verbally, political, physically, mentally or energetically. Of course the opposite is also true. To the degree to which we search for the humanity behind anyone's expression, we will inspire them to act more humanely toward us. Caring, compassion, empathy and nonviolent honesty are also boomerangs.

In order to have the presence, power and wisdom to send out only that which we want to receive back, we will need do our inner healing work and tune into a different part of our brains. This is the part that can be a receiver of the holographic intelligence of Gaia, the Goddess-Creatrix in Greek mythology. The "Gaia hypothesis" is both a scientific theory and a mass conscious reemergence of the ancient view of our Mother Earth as a living, pulsating, interconnected, intelligent, conscious whole. This unified intelligence of the universe understands the self-defeating nature of sawing off the tree branch on which we are sitting. When any group uses violence against any part of this whole conscious being, they are using violence against themselves. Therefore, regardless of the type of violence, coercion, and oppression we are seeking to transform, whether it be self-harshness and self-sacrifice, the domination/submission pattern of romantic relationships, or the hierarchical organization of groups, we will need to make a deep inner commitment to avoid using any kind of violence or coercion ourselves.

This is not as easy as it may sound. Nor is it easy to recognize when we are using subtly violent thinking, intentions and actions. Even those highly educated in the discipline of tolerance—leaders of the Civil Rights movement, those deeply committed to the spiritual principles of nonjudgment, and founders of the New Thought movement—all engage in the same judgmental, separateness-promoting, "anti-" speech and thought, without noticing its misalignment with their own principles. I assume that I, too, have some lingering habits of violence that I haven't yet noticed.

At a recent conference given by the Institute for Noetic Sciences and the Association for Global New Thought, Marianne Williamson shocked the audience by announcing that she had recently discovered she was a "hawk." (The dictionary defines this as "one who takes a militant attitude and advocates immediate vigorous action; *especially: a supporter of a war or warlike policy.*") It was surprising to hear this statement coming from the mouth of the world's leading teacher of the *Course in Miracles* (which says that love is the only answer, and all communication is either a call for love or an offering of love), best-selling author of *A Return to Love,* a leader in the creation of a Department of Peace in our government and an advocate for Dennis Kucinich's presidential candidacy. She is truly one of the world's best-known proponents of love and peace, yet she had spoken about certain people (like George W. Bush) in hawkish, adversarial, judgmental and therefore violent ways. It took a great deal of courage and consciousness on her part to acknowledge that in front of hundreds of her colleagues, and to attest to her own need to grow into a more evolved, integrated consciousness. Marianne went on to create a very empowering, loving workshop experience at the conference. I was especially pleased that she invited me to play the song "Bridges of Love" by Stephen Longfellow Fisk, allowed me to pass out copies of the book *Nonviolent Communication* to the hundreds of participants, and said, "As far as spiritually conscious social activism goes, Marshall Rosenberg is it!"

It is tempting to think of the other as "wrong" and to start carrying enemy images of those "hateful, violent" other people when we "know" we are "right" and righteous. It is particularly easy to delude ourselves when we have a gang to support us in our forceful thoughts and actions, whether they be right wing or left. Marianne went on to explain how acknowledging her hawkishness was allowing her to transcend it and embrace a power much more powerful than forcefulness, violence or righteous judgment.

I like the way David R. Hawkins, M.D., Ph.D., talks about the difference between power and force in his excellent book *Power v. Force:*

> Force always moves against something, whereas power doesn't move against anything at all. Force is incomplete and therefore has to be fed energy constantly. Power is total and complete in itself and requires nothing from outside. It makes

no demands; it has no needs. Because force has an insatiable appetite, it constantly consumes. Power, in contrast, energizes, gives forth, supplies, and supports. Power gives life and energy — force takes these away. We notice that power is associated with compassion and makes us feel positively about ourselves. Force is associated with judgment and makes us feel poorly about ourselves.

This is why a lot of peace activism is so ineffective. Activists often do not feel good about themselves. They feel angry and powerless, which attracts more angry powerless people to them. And then they have lifeless meetings where the most controlling, angriest people eventually take all the leadership positions. Jean Houston was right when she said that in order for the peace movement to be successful, we have to learn how to make peace *sexy*. In other words: powerful, loving, holistic and embracing all parts of ourselves and our world.

Without a certain spiritual clarity and commitment, we will very likely be sucked into the same system of pseudo-righteous Dominator thinking that we are trying to change. As Goethe once wrote, "Until one is committed, there is hesitancy, the chance to draw back, always ineffectiveness. The moment one definitely commits oneself, then Providence moves too." From the world of psychology the mystical Carl Jung wrote, "You always become the thing you fight the most," and from philosopher Friedrich Nietzsche comes, "Whoever fights monsters should see to it that in the process he does not become a monster." Wink seems to be expressing this "violence as boomerang" idea when he writes,

> Reality appears to be so constructed, whether physically or spiritually, that every action creates an equal and opposite reaction. Thus every attempt to fight the Domination System by dominating means is destined to result in domination. When we resist evil with evil, when we lash out at it in kind, we simply guarantee its perpetuation, as we ourselves are made over into its likeness. The way of nonviolence, the way Jesus chose, is the only way that is able to overcome evil with-

out creating new forms of evil and making us evil in turn. To those trapped in the Myth of Redemptive Violence (which is a type of spiritual militarism, and the myth of choice for Marxists, fascists, Nazis, capitalists, atheists and certain churchgoers alike), nonviolence must appear suicidal. But to those who have looked unflinchingly at the record of violence in the everyday world, nonviolence appears to be the only way left. And not just for Christians; for the world.

Even if we have decided to use violence or coercion only as a last resort, taking this position may well prevent us from tapping our own well of creativity and compassion when it is really needed. Walter Wink writes,

> Faith requires at times marching into the waters before they part (Josh. 3:15-16). Those who have not committed themselves to nonviolence in advance and under all circumstances are less likely to discover the creative nonviolent option in the desperate urgency of a crisis. They are already groping for the trigger, just when they should be praying and improvising. It may be that only an unconditional renunciation of violence can concentrate our minds sufficiently to find a nonviolent response when the crisis comes.

This concentration of our minds and attunement to the big picture and long range consequences can be a spiritual practice and an act of manifestation. Call it holistic selfishness, holographic intelligence, ecological awareness, supra-emotional intelligence, an intuitive interrelationship with universal intelligence, *ahimsa* (Gandhi's term for a spiritual consciousness of nonviolence), or just plain common sense, it is something we must consciously choose, lest we fall back on the de*fault* setting of our cultural training. This default setting finds fault somewhere and then justifies the use of violence, coercion or oppression.

But what is this *ahimsa?* Is it what I was taught in Sunday school? I learned that Jesus said to always love one another, which meant be *nice,* translate be passive, no matter what the other person was doing.

We were quoted the scripture, chapter and verse about how Jesus said we were no longer to live "an eye for and eye and a tooth for a tooth" because we were supposed to "not resist an evil doer" but instead if someone hits us on our right cheek, we should turn the other cheek, etc.

Forty years of my life passed before I found out that this translation of the bible was just King James's version. According to Wink, King James did not want anyone thinking they had any option except submission to a sovereign's policies. The Scholars Version of the Bible does not say to not resist evil (my translation would be someone who is acting violently toward you) but "Do not retaliate against violence with violence." What a difference! And of course it makes historical sense because Jesus' whole life is a lesson in civil disobedience resisting the "Evil Roman Empire." And it makes schoolyard sense. To just be passive and let schoolyard bullies use you as target practice to help them develop their "bad reputation" is dangerous and deeply humiliating. And to try to fight them physically is to enter their battlefield, a sort of suicide by bully. But Jesus rejected both passivity and violence. He was offering an out, what Wink calls "the third way." This third way did not involve violence but a way to equalize power, status and the playing field.

To really understand this, one needs to understand the Bible in its social context. When Jesus said "If any one strikes you on the right cheek, turn to him the other also," there is a cultural importance to his saying the "right" cheek. This is because in this right-handed world to hit someone on the right cheek with your right hand you would have to be back handing them. And in Jesus' culture at the time there were great penalties for gesturing at, or hitting someone with your "unclean" (translate toilet) hand. So this striking was really about insulting or humiliating someone to put them back in their place, not a fight between peers. It was also illegal at the time for a peer to hit a peer. Jesus was preaching to the downtrodden, those who were being oppressed by the government and the androcratic (male dominated) culture. This humiliating, status quo preserving, backhanding occurred between a master and a slave, parent and a child, men and women.

When the oppressed person turns the other cheek toward the oppressor, the oppressor can no longer backhand him. If he tried to backhand him again he would have to hit him square in the nose. And of course the left hand was not an option. This turning of the other cheek effectively makes the statement, "I refuse to give you the power to humiliate me. I am your equal."

This same spirit of nonviolent resistance permeated other advice Jesus gave. He told his followers that if someone sues you for your outer garment give him also your inner garment. According to Jewish law this would create a situation where the creditor would be standing there in court with all the clothes leaving the debtor naked. This would be terribly embarrassing for the creditor.

And when Jesus suggests that if a Roman soldier asks you to carry his pack one mile, carry it two, he is empowering the oppressed citizen to take the initiative and turn the tables. The image of the soldier asking the citizen to please give his pack back was at the time, empowering, exhilarating and hilarious. No wonder they praised him as their savior.

So Jesus not only taught his disciples to love their enemies compassionately but also to passionately stand up to them. It was an early version of what Swami Beyondananda calls "Absurdiveness Training" where we are reminded "Don't get even, get odd!" I too have been teaching and practicing this profound aikido-like Marshall Rosenberg Art, I sometimes call tongue fu. Sometimes I give play shops in "Conflict Improv" because it helps keep me keep my "Clown Chakra" open.

My four year old daughter Mataya gave me an example of this when she was playing in a garden near a neighbor's house. I was unaware of it but the neighbor was really getting frustrated about Mataya refusing to leave the neighbor's garden. Finally the neighbor got very angry, forcibly grabbed Mataya and removed her. Mataya's response was "Wheeeeee! That was fun!"

Another time while playing basketball, a man got really angry at something I did and began to stick his face into my face. At first my ego responded as I got scared and angry and stuck my nose against his, like men do when they are about to fight. A flash of creative intuition told me to just kiss him, and I did. He was disgusted and began to spit and wipe his face, but it did prevent a fight.

Of course we need to be careful not to use any of these techniques of nonviolent resistance to humiliate or take revenge. They can however be helpful in avoiding the dark side of peace loving philosophies and organizations, which is to be self-sacrificing, nice and martyristic. We can learn to be so sentimentally empathetic that we allow others to get their needs met at our expense and think we are being spiritual. I know this is what I learned in Sunday school.

I wonder if the statute of limitations has run out and it is too late to sue. In the name or restorative justice I would love to get some kind of compensation for what it has cost me to believe that being nice was being holy. And while I am feeling litigious, I wonder if I could become Jesus' libel lawyer and sue some of the preachers out there for libel and defamation of character. When they claim that Jesus was telling us "not to resist evil" by being passive, and to always return some kind of ill defined, airy fairy love for hate, that is not what he lived or said. It is such an impractical idealism that it turns people off, especially young people, to the power of a holistic Higher Self Centered love that can protect us. Jesus' love was uncompromising and unconditional but it was not, and he was not, *nice.* He was REAL. I would not sue for revenge but just to set the record straight, rescue Jesus' maligned name and to protect future victims from living a humiliating, painful shallow life of pseudo-spirituality.

Being REAL is about holding a fierce loving compassionate connection to ourselves as we confront those who would express violence of word, action or energy toward us. It is about maintaining that eye of the hurricane focus on the wholeness that contains both the other and I. From this grounded connection I have no fear of what the other may say or do, as all my attention is absorbed in my intention to respond with strength and compassion for both of us.

Where we choose to focus our attention determines the kind of world we create for ourselves today, and for our children tomorrow. This training of one's attention involves establishing an empathic connection to the need behind the deed. By this I mean that whatever strategy of violence or evil we are confronted with, we must first receive whatever empathy we need to deal with the pain that has been created in us. Then we may focus our empathy on the persons who did the violence until we achieve the penetrating spiritual insight required to connect with the human need expressed through the deed. We then can see that, given their training in Dominator thinking, this is the only strategy they could have thought of to get their needs met. Once we have this empathic, non-judgmental connection with the person, we have great power to influence and educate them in ways of meeting their needs that are not at the expense of others' needs.

These principles of reconciliation are not only true on the local or personal level. They are also applicable on the global political levels. I think it is very important to remember this as we consider how we want to respond to the tragedies of 9-11. It is our human ignorance and lack of faith that results in our use of violence. Let us take responsibility for our violence, compassionately understand and forgive ourselves for it, but then do the inner work and education it takes to be prepared to act more powerfully and nonviolently in the future.

As long as we keep justifying our violence, we blind ourselves to the need to find a more creative, powerful way to restore safety and harmony. We might justify our individual violence by thinking "I had no choice," "they were violent first," "they deserved my violence," "they made me mad," or "I lost control and it just happened." As a collective, we might claim, "we had no choice," "they struck at us first," "we are just protecting ourselves," "God is on our side and wants this war," "they are bad people and will not listen to reason," or "this is a just war." Whatever our justifications, we will still have to cope with the loss of internal integrity and the external escalation and/or other destructive consequences. Wink provides a unique Christian perspective on how and why nations justify their acts of violence when he writes,

> A nation may feel that it must fight in order to prevent an even greater evil. But that does not cause the lesser evil to cease being evil. Declaring a war "just" is simply a ruse to rid ourselves of guilt. But we can no more free ourselves of guilt by decree than we can declare ourselves forgiven by fiat. If we have killed, it is a sin, and only God can forgive us, not a propaganda apparatus that declares our dirty wars "just".
>
> Governments and guerrilla chiefs are not endowed with the power to absolve us from sin. Only God can do that. And God is not mocked. The whole discussion of "just" wars is sub-Christian.

So whether you call it a jihad, the Arabic word for "holy war," or use the Western term "just war," the intent to justify the violence is the same.

Sometimes the hypocrisy expressed by governments, churches and institutional leaders is so extreme that it becomes comical to me. When I was in Northern Ireland working with mixed groups of Protestants and Catholics, it was tragic but also funny to hear how they talked about each other. First Protestant leaders would condemn the violent actions of Catholic militia groups, and Catholic leaders would condemn the violence of Protestant militia groups. Then both Catholic and Protestant leaders would praise the heroic, Biblically justified actions of their own freedom fighting militiamen, assuring their place in heaven.

This kind of macabre humor occasionally reaches new depths in shallowness thru satire on American TV. One of my favorite TV shows as a kid was "Get Smart" (which Wink also writes about) where the inept arrogant spy Maxwell Smart was engaged in a mythic struggle to defeat the forces of evil known as Chaos. Max worked for the good guys of the agency called Control. Once after a particularly brutal killing of one of the bad guy agents from Chaos by the good guys from Control, Agent 99, Max's partner, asked something like, "Gosh Max I sure wish we had another way besides killing and hurting people. Sometimes I think we are no better than they are." To which Max responded in his dry sardonic way, "99, of course we have to kill and hurt people; that's how we preserve everything that's good in the world."

When we dehumanize a group of people by pinning a demonizing label on them like "terrorist," we set into motion the psychological dynamics that allow us to treat them as less than human and exterminate them. We deny that God has the power to transform these particular people into loving human beings again. We play God by suggesting that God is not within them, and therefore they deserve our punishment.

I have heard President George W. Bush suggest that the only thing Saddam Hussein and the terrorists understand is military force, and they cannot be reasoned with because they hate us. This of course is the same argument those often called "terrorists" taught in their training camps to justify their violent tactics against the U.S. The idea that our "enemies" have to achieve a certain level of moral development or reasoning before we can engage them nonviolently does not hold true historically and is one of the most commonly used political tricks to justify genocide, violence and oppression. Those who are suggesting we must use violence against certain peoples because they are racist and violent are using the very thinking they are condemning. Nazis claimed the Jews were less than human and the KKK say blacks are subhuman and many in our present government suggest that they people they have labeled "terrorist" do not have the capacity for human interaction. Jesus did not wait for the Roman soldiers to start going to Sunday school before he engaged them with his teachings of nonviolent resistance. No, he knew they were human, despite the violent thinking they were caught up in. He trusted God to have the power to transform them. How can someone call themselves a follower of Christ and then suggest some of God's children cannot be forgiven or redeemed and need to be killed?

And as we continue to use our resources to kill and punish people, we will soon run out of resources to protect people. What we fear we draw near. Why?

Dr. Hawkins explains:

> Force always creates counterforce; its effect is to polarize rather than unify. Polarization always implies conflict; its cost, therefore, is always high. Because force incites polarization, it inevitably produces a win/lose dichotomy; and because somebody always loses, enemies are created. Constantly faced with enemies, force requires constant defense. Defensiveness is invariably costly, whether in the marketplace, politics, or international affairs.

And, I would add, also in personal relationships.

But what to do instead?

Marshall Rosenberg responded this way right after 9-11:

> Peace in the Middle East requires something far more difficult than revenge or merely turning the other cheek; it requires empathizing with the fears and unmet needs that provide the impetus for people to attack each other. Being aware of these feelings and needs, people have no desire to attack back because they can see the human ignorance leading to these attacks; instead, their goal becomes providing the empathic connection and education which will enable them to transcend their violence and engage in cooperative relationships.

Empathy Has No Enemy

I was once dramatically confronted with the life-or-death necessity of making such a choice. I and my partner Debbie, our daughter who was then one year old, and a friend of ours named Amy were sitting on a couch, holding hands, laughing and talking. It was Thanksgiving. Amy's ex-partner, Steve was also visiting from out of town. Several times we had invited Steve to come over and join us on the couch, but he chose instead to sit in the hallway on the floor, slumped over. He had a pained look on his face, and occasionally he muttered something under his breath.

After some time, we were feeling frustrated and distracted, so I asked Steve, "I am feeling really uncomfortable with you out there suffering in the hallway. I would like us all to be together. Would you be willing to either join us and tell us what is going on with you, or go into the other room?" This was just the spark the powder keg needed. Steve got up in a huff and ran into the kitchen and began rummaging around in a drawer. Then he came around the corner into the living room where we were all still sitting, waving a knife. He threatened to hurt Amy, me, Debbie, and our daughter. I later learned that Steve had been working himself up into a jealous rage about the attention Debbie and I were showing Amy. He had been wanting to reestablish a connection with Amy, but she was no longer willing to deal with his mood swings, depression, anger and dominating control. So when Steve saw us all having the kind of caring connection that he so desperately wanted, it triggered his comparison shame jackal ("I must be worth less than these other people to Amy") and also a deep insecurity about being loved, which he covered over with an intense, compulsive, angry need for control.

When Steve appeared with the knife, I was in shock, but I tried to appear reasonable and unafraid. But then my daughter got frightened and began to cry. This seemed to really irritate Steve, who took a step in her direction.

Suddenly time slowed way, way down. I entered what felt like a surreal, slow-motion movie, in which there was all the time in the world to think about what to do next. I found myself standing up from the couch, my belly filling with rage, my arm cocking back, and my hand making a fist. I remember enjoying the rush of adrenaline and the conversion from fear and powerlessness to an exhilarating, powerful rage. I felt almighty and Godlike in my absolute righteousness.

I had no doubt that I could knock Steve out. And who would blame me? No one! Everyone would agree that I had a perfect right, in fact a responsibility to my defenseless daughter, to protect her by any means necessary. My righteous rage echoed the myth of redemptive violence, the idea that there is good violence, and it is a form of spirituality.

Then my mind expanded its intelligence. I considered humankind's history of the use of violence to combat violence. I had come to an evolutionary fork in the road, and I had to choose. I was just about to swing when a whimper came from Mataya. I imagined her saying, "Daddy don't. Even if you solve this problem this way think of what kind of world you will be creating for me in the future." It was as though the universal intelligence of Gaia herself were speaking to me. I flashed forward to see the domino effect of my violence creating an ever more dangerous world for my daughter. Once I was clear about the consequences of taking any action based on my violent cultural programming, a spirit of knowing entered me and began to direct the show. I began to feel the "peace that passeth all understanding" as my heart welled up with the emotion of compassion.

I relaxed my arm, opened my hand and turned my eyes calmly toward Steve's face. As my heart opened toward him, I felt a rush of empathy for his anguish. I could feel the energy of empathy weaving us into one. As I felt what was going on inside his emotional body, all images of, "attacker," "enemy," and "madman" melted away. In that moment a phrase entered my mind, "empathy has no enemy," and I understood what it meant. Only the illusion of our separateness can allow for the appearance of an attack. I felt great gratitude to myself for the empathy I had received and given to those inner shadow parts of myself. This work allowed me to feel the compassion for Steve I would have wished for myself. All that I saw before me was a desperately hurting, tortured soul.

As I was able to connect with that in him, I felt safe and no longer at odds with him. I had the most amazing feeling that I *was* him and that he was not a threat to me. He looked at my face for just a moment, grimaced as if in agony and then began screaming at me, "I am in control here. You want me to show you control. I will show you who is in control." Suddenly and violently he raised the knife above his head and plunged the blade into his own forearm about two inches deep.

I felt a surge of compassion for his physical pain, as well as his anger, shame and angst. As I felt this connection, all fear left my body. I started to slowly walk toward him with my arms out, and with tears in my eyes I looked into his eyes. Just as I got up to him he turned away from me. I gently wrapped my arms around him from behind, empathetically feeling his pain, and said with true caring, "Your pain is my pain and your wounds are my wounds." He started to sob in my arms, and wipe blood onto his face. I took a towel and wrapped his arm up to slow the bleeding. For that moment I knew what it was like to be the face of love and to see no enemy. I experienced the safety of becoming one with the "enemy," leaving no-one else for him to attack.

Creating Compassionate Culture

As we set out to re-create ourselves and our culture, let us always stay aware of the divine harmony that already exists between our passion for ourselves and our compassion for others. Understanding this awakens a sense of connection with our community (common-unity) that eliminates anger, hate, isolation and insignificance as well as providing a greater opportunity for the realization of autonomy, self-expression, intimacy, safety and spiritual intoxication. This intoxication perhaps can only be understood by those who have gone beyond ego boundaries and had the resulting peak experience. One reason we experience bliss and euphoria as we open up to nonviolent community is because, as Wink writes, "Nonviolence is not just a means to the realm of God. It is a quality of that realm itself."

In this process of self-development and creation of community, we must first be careful not to fall back on the Dominator, jackal patterns of relating from our past. We must practice gentleness and compassion for our own dominating self-harshness. We must make a clear commitment to never indulge in sneaky coercion or overt intimidation of others, but seek instead to penetrate through the layers of pain and confusion to the human needs that human beings are always expressing and that we all share. We must value ourselves through self-responsible assertive honesty with others, reaching for that quality of connection that inevitability leads to everyone getting their needs met.

The Patriarchy is Passing

I sit in shock at my computer today April 22nd, 2002. My father died yesterday, at 5:30 AM, on April 21st, at the Veterans Hospital in Phoenix, Arizona. Thomas Bryson was a World War II veteran, mean as a snake — the harsh, totalitarian patriarch of the family. Had I grown up with him, I imagine I would have hated him, as some of his other sons do. But as I was put in foster homes early on, I only knew the part of him that loved to wrestle with little five-year-old boys. And that part was gentle, playful and loved my life force.

What happened to that sweet gentle soul, to turn it into a monster? It got swept up into a fear-based social vortex. He became a part of that system and served its purposes. It destroyed him, body, mind and spirit. This is also what has happened to so much of humankind on our planet. Now that my father has passed, I am one of the elders of my family, with no abandoning father to blame for my personal problems, no abusive patriarch to hold responsible for all the social ills. Now I truly must quit whining about the story of my life and the world as it is. (My publicist said to me, "Look, if you don't like the headlines, go out and make some new ones!") Now I choose to drop the storybook sword of my victimhood and pick up the pen to write a new story that no longer elevates men, might and spirituality over women, nature and sexuality.

The new story I write is not a myth of redemptive violence. It is a parable of humane potential. It is not a Passion Play of pain and death, but a compassion play of pleasure and life. Its characters step down from the hierarchy of Jacob's Ladder and join a level, egalitarian Sara's Circle. I tie myself to the mast of the nonviolent partnership principles I would instill in others, lest I get swept up into the prevailing winds of the typhoon of tyranny. Stephen Longfellow Fisk sings it this way in his song "Bridges of Love":

If we can build great bridges across the mighty waves between distant ridges,

Is it a task, too great, to build a bridge across the depths of hate?

If we can reach so far to send men up to the moon and rockets to the stars,

Why are we still so far apart?

Why can't we find a way from soul to soul, from heart to heart?

Bridges of steel reach from shore to shore, bridges of love reach so much more.

They link our common hopes, our common ground, joining one and all the whole world round.

We can all build bridges of love each day, with our eyes, our smiles, our touch, our will to find a way.

There is no distance we cannot span, the vision is in our hearts.

The power is in our hands.

For now more than ever what the world needs more of, is to reach, to reach for each other with bridges of love.

A name for one of these bridges is compassion. Schmookler writes, "In addition to trust, another foundation for the bridges between people is compassion, the ability to identify emotionally with the experience of others. The ability to place oneself sympathetically in another's shoes is, after all, the psychological prerequisite of the Golden Rule: do unto others as you would have them do unto you." But he continues, "We cannot have compassion for (feeling with) others if we kill off feeling within ourselves. The capacity to embrace our own true emotions is conversely a prerequisite of our being able truly to allow others into our hearts."

Compassion is an essential element to having love in our lives. David Hawkins also suggests it is the key to physical health: "Once we really understand the human condition, we'll feel compassion where we once might have felt condemnation. Compassion is one of the highest of all of the energy attractor power patterns. Our capacity to understand, forgive, and accept is directly linked to our personal health."

The path to peace takes courage. But which kind of courage? Is it the controlling courage of righteous rage that keeps us up in the "gun towers" of our heads, forever ranting and raving about who is right and wrong? Or is it the courage of our hearts that allows us to come down into our bodies to risk connecting and conflicting as we create conscious community?

Here are some guiding principles for a nonviolent community and a new culture as offered by Dieter Duhm of the Zegg community (www.zegg.de) (with a slight modification for an American culture).

Twelve Theses for a Non-violent Culture

1. Home for the Children. In a non-violent world children grow up in confidence and trust. The future of humanity depends on the fate of its children. A childhood marked by distrust and violence will not produce humane beings. Provide a home to children where they can again trust their parents.

2. Love and Trust. Love is the source of humane thinking and non-violent action. Love comes from trust and trust comes from truth. Create living environments where human beings have no reason for lies and fear. Create the social and ecological conditions for love. Confidence and love are the most fundamental powers in all of creation.

3. Sexuality. Sexuality is an elementary force of life and of the joy of existence. Sexuality is autonomous. It can neither be controlled by patriarchal marriage pledges demanding obedience, nor by tight external moral constrictions; instead it needs truth and trust. Create the moral and social conditions for healthy sexuality.

4. Partnership. Partnership is the highest form of relationship. It has its roots in a common way of thinking. In no way is partnership in opposition to a consensus-based sexual morality, because it is itself free of jealousy. True partnership is the most radical model for a relationship between human beings that is free of violence and fear. Create the mental basis for a partnership free of jealousy.

5. Community. The organic environment for human beings is the community. Natural values like truth, trust, solidarity and responsible participation—without philosophical nit-picking—can only be realized within communities that have developed organically. The non-

violent society of human beings is a network of communities who value consensus and a common unity, and whose ultimate goal is a world where everyone's needs are met nonviolently. Only in this way can the original concept of socialism be brought to reality in a humane way. Create functioning communities.

6.   Freedom and Autonomy of the Individual. A free world comprises individuals who say what they think and share what touches them. They are not subordinate to anything but their own knowledge and consciousness. The mature community is a grassroots democracy of free individuals. It is a human collective that is not collectively led in the name of a leader or an ideology. The individual and the community are equal and complementary forces in a non-violent world.

7.   Thinking. The reflecting intellect is a young and powerful fruit on the tree of evolution. Free and creative thinking dissolves all rigid ideologies. The secrets of existence are beyond all scientific or religious terminology. Individual autonomy is a direct result of a thinking that is free of fear. Overcome all creeds and dogmas of scientific and political systems. Create universities for the powers of growth inherent in free thinking.

8.   Religion. Just like Eros and the intellect, spirituality is one of the elemental powers of human existence. We live in an endless radiant universe. Everything we are and everything surrounding us has roots in the universe. Spiritual love is the connectedness with the whole. Therefore we do not need a religious confession nor predetermined answers. The answer will come through the spiritual opening of the mind. Create a free religious spirit without laws and without dogmas.

9.   Nature. Nature is our link with creation. We are its offspring, like a child that is born from its mother's womb. The secret of human existence is part of the secret of nature. Whatever we do to nature we do to ourselves. The outer and inner environment are two aspects of the same world. Let us take care of Mother Nature and become aware of the processes of growth and their rhythms and interrelatedness.

Cooperation with all vital energies and respect for life are the prerequisites for a non-violent and humane civilization.

10. Animals. Stop all cruelty toward animals. Like us they are part of the living organism of the biosphere. Like us they are beings with souls, just at a different level of evolution. In a non-violent culture, whales are not killed, animals are not kept for slaughter, and fur farming does not exist. Create spaces for a coexistence of human beings and animals that is free of fear. Animals do not exist for us to slaughter but to help us to learn to see.

11. Biotopes for Healing. All of the thoughts above join together to form a new biotope for healing. Such a biotope contains the informational totality for a non-violent existence on planet Earth. Create pilot models for this informational totality. Create international centers where the social, technical, ecological and spiritual structures are such that the healing powers of life — trust, Eros, Logos and symbiosis — are promoted in the best possible way.

12. Networks of Human Beings. Today, within all countries and cultures on earth, there are people who have irrevocably understood the necessity of a positive inner and outer revolution. They all contribute certain thoughts, certain convictions, and certain aspects to the overall view of the tasks at hand. It is not machines but people who decide if a future worth living is possible. In that spirit we want to invite you to join the network for a non-violent earth.

A Utopian Reality

I have heard of courageous people who risk their lives on Greenpeace boats, placing themselves between whalers' harpoons, and the whales they would protect. Some of them hate the whalers, in an unconscious attempt to work out their authority issues with these projections of their own patriarchal fathers and culture. Others, in the same boat, may have done more of their inner work. They are now answering the call of a real authority, one that compels them to protect and love the whales. I would ask us all to ask ourselves this question: Are we hating the whalers or loving the whales? If we are hating the whalers, we will become like whalers, contributing to the consciousness that allows humankind's domination of the earth and seas. If we do our inner healing work, then we can stay focused in our love for the whales, ourselves and Mother Earth. From this energy we can truly start creating conscious nonviolent partnership communities and relationships. Then we will not be afraid to realize our potential for power, for our souls will finally and truly trust our benevolent intentions.

Some people are tired of all the work involved in trying to save fundamentalists from their oppression of women, children and sexuality, as well as shape up the schools, convert corporate culture, and topple autocratic governments — all before breakfast. Lately I too have had much more passion for creating a new partnership culture and community for myself, my family and my close friends, rather than trying to change the old culture. I think there is a line in the Bible that says, "Don't put new wine into old wineskins."

I also believe that as people sense the clarity, warmth and respect being expressed through the members of these new partnership communities, those living in Dominator organizational systems will want to join. Maybe we don't have to tear down Dominator organizational systems. Maybe they will wither away from lack of interest.

If we create community systems that better meet peoples' needs for respect, acceptance, sexuality, closeness, giving, gender equality, emotional safety, empathy, celebration, warmth, and support, perhaps people will simply quit participating in Dominator organizations. Perhaps they will quit putting time and money into their Dominator churches and clubs, their dysfunctional school systems and governments controlled by old boy networks. The Nobel Prize winner and discoverer of the polio vaccine, Jonas Salk, wrote in his book *Anatomy of Reality* that a new culture will evolve through a new science of empathy based on both reason and intuition "to bring about a change in the collective mind that will constructively influence the course of the human future." I believe many people are itching to involve themselves in viable alternative partnership communities. Peoples' souls are longing for a place to contribute their gifts, to play with others who are really fun, to create schools with people who share more humane values and, live with those who are more alive.

Creating Your Own Compassionate Community

A conscious community is the best resource anyone can have, particularly for growth and joy. As psychiatrist Jean Baker Miller writes, "[the longing for community] allows for the emergence of the truth: that for everyone—men as well as women—individual development proceeds only by means of affiliation." If you do not have one, you can cocreate one with your friends. I just started inviting my friends and their friends to do some of the following activities, and gradually the need to become more organized so we could enjoy even more community spirit experience arose. Here are some examples from "Communities" magazine (www.ic.org) of the kinds of activities that form the "glue" needed for community building:

1. Personal sharing time.

2. Conflict resolution time.

4. Shared meals.

4. Decision-making that includes everyone.

5. Children in the community.

6. Shared values, a common vision and purpose.

7. Appreciating and acknowledging each other.

8. Singing, dancing, making music.

9. Celebrations and rituals.

10. Snuggling, puppy piles.

11. Creating theatrical performances.

12. Cocreating projects like a newsletter or event.

13. Working together on projects that serve not only the community but the environment, the city, the country, the world.

What I am writing about is not a nice utopian dream, because it is already happening in many places around the world. Besides the

Human Awareness Institute communities, NVC communities, and New Thought churches, there are many, many other evolving conscious organizations. Of course the communities that are the strongest are the ones that emerge organically, without a charismatic leader or school of philosophy or religion, as this often leads to endless nit-picking about what is or is not correct. On another level, there is a new community that does not exist. It is awakened within the heart, through the quality of connection we make with the real people in our lives. It rises up in our hearts when our compassion for the suffering of the world is touched. This new community is invisible. But it shows itself through your eyes, your touch, your words, and your actions.

The Author and His Work

WWW.LANGUAGEOFCOMPASSION.COM

Kelly Bryson, MA, MFT, is an "edu-tainer": a speaker, author, life/career coach, humorist, singer, poet, workshop leader, mediator, and a licensed psychotherapist. He has trained with John Bradshaw, Ram Dass, Albert Ellis, Rollo May, Virginia Satir, Gerry Jampolsky, Jean Houston, and Marshall Rosenberg. He has been an authorized trainer for the international Center for Nonviolent Communication for twenty years, and has trained thousands in the US., Europe and the Middle East including hot spots like Croatia, Serbia., Northern Ireland and Israel. He trains and consults with corporations (Paul Mitchell Salons, Tony Robbins Research), churches, schools (Body Mind College), universities, (University of California Long Beach) and organizations (Institute of Noetic Science). He speaks for all sorts of gatherings, keynotes at conventions, and has appeared on numerous television (like NBC-TV San Francisco) and radio shows (KPBS and KPFA in Los Angeles). He has written for and been featured in many publications including Elle magazine.

Kelly Bryson grew up in several different foster homes and was exposed to several very different family systems. The confusion that resulted started him on a lifelong journey to find clarity, love, meaning, harmony and truth. He enrolled in the Psychology program of the

University of Florida in 1970, studying The Transparent Self with Sidney Jourard. He experimented with psychedelic drugs, then joined an Indian Ashram community and practiced celibacy, selfless service, Eastern meditation and spirituality for twelve years.

When he discovered that he could not transcend the earth plane, he left the ashram and took the job of managing a restaurant near Disney World. He took a graduate humanistic psychology course at the University of West Georgia where he studied the phenomenology of his own inner experience, among other things. It was here that he met Dr. Marshall Rosenberg and soon after started teaching Nonviolent Communication to adolescents and their families in the treatment centers where he worked. He moved to San Diego in 1984 where he studied with Virginia Satir, became a licensed psychotherapist, started a private practice and founded the Center for Compassion.

Nonviolent Communication Santa Cruz (NVCSC)

Kelly Bryson has collaborated with the founders of Compassionate Communication Santa Cruz, Jean Morrison and Christine King, along with Rick and Aviva Longinotti, to create a not-for-profit organization called Nonviolent Communication of Santa Cruz (NVCSC). Working together, this group has established the Center for Compassion, which houses group training rooms and offices. Serving Santa Cruz, South Bay and the Central Coast of California, NVCSC supports the mission of the international Center for Nonviolent Communication (www.cnvc.org) — by assisting individuals, couples, organizations and groups in learning lifelong skills for communicating with compassion, sharing resources, and resolving conflicts through:

- Monthly introductory talks
- Full and half day workshops
- Audio/video presentations
- Practice and book study groups
- Conflict mediation
- Workshops for specific workplace, school, and church groups

Website: www.NVCSantaCruz.org
Email us at ccsc@baymoon.com or call 831-425-3055
Kelly Bryson, in collaboration with the NVCSC team, also provides:

Services and Training for Individuals, Couples and Families:

Weekly Practice/Support/Growth Groups
Various weekend and longer Intensive trainings
Private sessions for marital, individual or family counseling for most issues.
Phone therapy, Life/Career Coaching, consulting, counseling.
Because Kelly Bryson MFT is a licensed psychotherapist, he can accept payment from most health insurances for sessions, classes and trainings.

Services and Training for Businesses, Churches (all flavors) and any Organization

- Basic skills Introductory presentation
- Tailor-made Skills Training Program (based on the most frequently encountered on-the-job real-life communication challenges.)
- Conflict Resolution Training and Services (as alternative to litigation)
- Customer Relations Training
- Team Building
- Custom Designed Organizational Development Program

Communicating with self responsible honesty and empathy is the basis of all successful collaboration. Hurt Feelings Hurt Business. So cultivate a culture of honesty and compassion, make it safe to bring your full passionate selves to work by getting NVC into your organization!

Communi-Team Building

- Start a Compassionate Community from scratch
- Grow Compassion and Consciousness in an existing community
- Heal old hurts and conflicts in your present community or organization
- Develop Nonviolent Communication skills in your group or business.

Call Kelly to book a Speaking Engagement:

The following are some of Kelly's speaking titles. He has also has given many Sunday Morning "Sermons" for churches of various denominations.

Don't be Nice, Be Real!—Balancing Passion for Self with Compassion for Others

Nonviolent Communication—The Lost Language of Humanity; Empathy has no Enemy

Compassion vs. Coercion

The Power of Innocence

Twenty-first Century Relationships

Being Me and Loving You; Celebrating your Selfullness

Promote Power—Forget Force

Everyday Passion

Passionate Creating

Life Enriching Education

How stay Nonviolent in a Violent World!

How to Parent without Punishment (Or Rewards!)

How to stay Fearless in a Fearful World

There's no such thing as a happy ending to a miserable journey!

The Soulful Meaning of Money

Got Compassion?

About Money:

We wish to nurture an economy based upon the life-affirming value of giving and receiving from the heart. Therefore, we wish to make services and trainings available by donation. We do not receive any foundation support or grants, but do wish to contribute to a more just and compassionate world. Your donations allow us to make Nonviolent Communication Training available to those who need it regardless of their ability to pay. Also, they help to finance the international Center for Nonviolent Communication (now in 40 countries with over 150 authorized trainers) to do its healing work in Africa, Asia, the Middle East, South America and third world or war torn countries.

Resources

The Center for Nonviolent Communication (CNVC)

The NVC model was developed and refined over a period of thirty-five years by Marshall Rosenberg. Growing up Jewish in a turbulent and anti-Semitic Detroit neighborhood, Dr. Rosenberg developed a keen interest in conflict resolution and new forms of communication that would provide peaceful alternatives to the violence he encountered. His interest eventually led to graduate school, where he earned a Ph.D. in clinical psychology. But he was dissatisfied with the focus he saw there on pathology, which did not help him understand the very compassionate people he had also known. Further study of comparative religion, and his own varied life experience, convinced him that human beings are not inherently violent and motivated him to develop NVC. In 1984 he founded the Center for Nonviolent Communication (CNVC) a 501(c)3 organization and, in 1999, published his book *Nonviolent Communication: A Language of Compassion* (Puddle Dancer Press).

The Center for Nonviolent Communication is now a global organization whose vision is a world where everyone's needs are met peacefully. The mission of CNVC staff, trainers and volunteers is to contribute to this vision by facilitating the creation of life-serving systems within themselves, inter-personally, and within organizations. They do this by living and teaching the process of Nonviolent Communication (NVC), which strengthens the ability of people to compassionately connect with themselves and one another, share resources, and resolve conflicts.

NVC is a powerful process for inspiring compassionate connection and action. It provides a framework and set of skills to address all of these problems, from the most intimate relationships to global political conflicts. NVC can help prevent conflicts as well as peacefully resolve them. For many years the Center for Nonviolent Communication has been quietly contributing to a vast social transformation in thinking, speaking and acting, showing people how to connect with the life in themselves and others in ways that inspire a compassionate response.

NVC trainers are available to help organize workshops, participate in practice groups, and coordinate team building:

Center for Nonviolent Communication
2428 Foothill Blvd., Suite E
La Crescenta, CA 91214
Phone: (818) 957-9393; Fax; (818) 957-1424
E-mail: cnvc@cnvc.org
Website: www.cnvc.org

The Human Awareness Institute (HAI)

Love, intimacy and sexuality can be the hardest issues to deal with in a relationship. Human Awareness Institute workshops offer the skills that help people deal with these sensitive topics in their relationships. For many people, sexuality is a taboo subject. HAI offers a forum to learn, share our fears about and discuss intimate relationships. Workshops are specifically structured to provide a safe environment. HAI helps the individual define what love, intimacy and sexuality means to them, and in turn, how that affects the other areas of their life. HAI was founded in 1968 by Dr. Stan Dale. For over thirty years HAI has offered workshops dealing with intimate relationships and human sexuality. Over 50,000 people have participated.

The Human Awareness Institute
Phone: (800) 800 4117 Fax: (650) 593-3352
International: +1 650-571-5524
E-mail: office@hai.org
Web Site: www.hai.org

The Center for Partnership Studies

Partnership is a commitment to a way of living. It is a way of life based on harmony with nature, nonviolence, and gender, racial, and economic equity. During much of our prehistory, humanity was rooted in the partnership model. This is our lost heritage. Through a cultural shift, history became the familiar tale of violence, injustice, and domination. We need to restore our Earth and renew our communities. We need social and economic inventions based on partnership. This is the mission of the Center for Partnership Studies, and the life's work of celebrated author, Riane Eisler.

P.O. Box 30538
Tucson, AZ 85751
Phone: (520) 546-0176 Fax: (520) 546-2053
E-mail: center@partnershipway.org
Web Site: www.partnershipway.org

The Association for Global New Thought

The core purpose of the Association for Global New Thought is to consciously bring forth the evolving human and an awakened world through the practice of universal spiritual principles and the energy of unconditional love.

New Thought is a spiritually motivated way of life that embraces the ancient wisdom traditions of East and West. We embody the belief that consciousness is elementally creative, reciprocates thought, and thereby shapes all manifestation. Our principles reflect a universal conviction that the community of all life is sacred; our practices of meditation and prayer enhance a worldview promoting reverence for, and service to humanity and planet earth. New Thought is committed to global healing through personal transformation, community-building, interfaith, intercultural and interdisciplinary understanding and compassionate activism.

Phone: 805-563-7343
Website: www.agnt.org

Order Books:

Don't be Nice, Be Real By Kelly Bryson $15.00
The Places you could go, If you weren't Afraid of NO! By Kelly Bryson (An Adult/Kids Dr. Seuss-like poem book) $8.00
Rumi-nations By Kelly Bryson (One liners and short bursts of poetry, wisdom and humor) $8.00

Nonviolent Communication By Marshall Rosenberg $17.95
Life Enriching Education By Marshall Rosenberg $13.00
And many other great books Kelly recommends on his website.

CD's and Audio Tapes by Kelly

The Basic Steps to Nonviolent Communication . . . . .Tape-$10, CD-$15
A 90 minute production that simply, clearly maps out the steps to Nonviolent Communication Each step is defined, examples are given, role plays with Deb and Kelly are done and inspiring beautiful songs are sung to illustrate each principle.

Songs of Compassion (22 songs) . . . . .Tape-$10, CD-$15

A Spirituality named Compassion . . . . .Tape-$10, CD-$15
A great tape to introduce Nonviolent Communication to any new person. Kelly tells touching stories of how NVC was used, plays songs, and uses humor to a great audience.

Don't be Nice, Be Real—(2 tapes of radio interviews) . . . . . .Tapes-$20, CDs-$25
Kelly is interviewed about the underlying theories of NVC, listeners call and real life situations are worked with, plus many songs and stories.

Empathy has no Enemy . . . . .Tape-$10, CD-$15
How to love one's "Enemies" and how it is a path to safety and spiritual growth!

The Power of Innocence . . . . .Tape-$10, CD-$15
How to use NVC to heal fear, shame and guilt to uncover our ever present innocence. Kelly uses songs, stories and speech to teach how to use the *Power of that Innocence* to open ourselves to receiving loving connection and expressing creativity.

Speaking Peace—Two CD/tapes by Marshal Rosenberg ..Tapes-$20, CDs-$25
(NEW CD's!) By Dr. Rosenberg: *"Giraffe Fuel for Life,"* *"Needs and Empathy,"* *"Creating a Life-Serving System within Oneself,"* *"Intimate Relationships,"* *"Experiencing Needs as Gifts"* . . . .$15 ea.
Considerable discounts are given for quantities of all materials.

To Order any of the above, to contact Kelly, or get info about his schedule:

Go to website: www.LanguageOfCompassion.com. There are many other books, tapes, CD's, workbooks, videos and materials available for sale on the website.

Call Toll Free Phone 1-877-No-FEARS (663-3277) to order or:

Email—Kelly@LanguageOfCompassion.com with MasterCard or Visa number, name and expiration date

Or Make Checks payable to Kelly Bryson and mail to address on Website.

Please include $2.00 postage for each item purchased + California. tax. (7.5 cents per dollar).